Applying the Therapeutic Function of Professional Supervision

This book brings a fresh approach and conversation to the practice of professional supervision for human services by specifically articulating its often performed, but unnamed and under-explored therapeutic function. The discussion of the therapeutic function is timely given the rising complexities in our world, and the increasing awareness of emotional impacts of human service work. These impacts include stress, distress, emotional labour, indirect trauma, and direct trauma.

Posing a challenge and invitation to supervisors to comfortably inhabit the therapeutic function of supervision to increase emotional support to workers, it places safe practice and worker wellbeing at the heart of supervision to enable high quality service delivery for often the most vulnerable in society. While underpinned by theory, it is written to be practically applied and is developed from a 'lived experience' perspective, offering a unique glimpse into actual practice.

By modelling one of the main aims of professional supervision, which is to facilitate and enable the integration of experience into learning and knowledge, it will be of interest to all practitioners across a broad range of human services, particularly both new and experienced supervisors.

Nicki Weld (PhD) is a senior lecturer in the University of Auckland Post Graduate Professional Supervision Programme, and a supervisor and educator in human services in Aotearoa, New Zealand. She is a registered social worker with research interests in supervision, courage, trauma, and child and family work.

Applying the Therapeutic Function of Professional Supervision

Attending to the Emotional Impacts of Human Service Work

Nicki Weld

FOREWORD BY GILLIAN RUCH

Routledge
Taylor & Francis Group
LONDON AND NEW YORK

Cover image: © Getty Images

First published 2023
by Routledge
4 Park Square, Milton Park, Abingdon, Oxon OX14 4RN

and by Routledge
605 Third Avenue, New York, NY 10158

Routledge is an imprint of the Taylor & Francis Group, an informa business

© 2023 **Nicki Weld**

British Library Cataloguing-in-Publication Data
A catalogue record for this book is available from the British Library

ISBN: 978-1-032-41637-3 (hbk)
ISBN: 978-1-032-41636-6 (pbk)
ISBN: 978-1-003-35903-6 (ebk)

DOI: 10.4324/9781003359036

Typeset in Sabon
by codeMantra

To those I have provided supervision to, and to the supervisors I have received supervision from – thank you.

Contents

List of figures   xi
List of tables   xiii
Foreword   xv

Introduction   1

1   Defining the therapeutic function of supervision   9
    Types of supervision 9
    Interdisciplinary supervision 13
    Roles in professional supervision 15
    The functions of professional supervision 18
    The therapeutic and therapy boundary 20
    Ethical considerations 26
    Summary 27

2   Relational skills to enable the therapeutic function   30
    Developing the supervisory relationship 30
    Presence 32
    Attuning 34
    Listening deeply 36
    Enabling vulnerability 37
    Cultural humility 39
    Summary 42

3   Developing a coherent narrative   45
    Reflective learning processes 46
    Explore inaccurate thoughts 49

Connect to strengths and existing resiliency 50
Moving forward 52
Summary 54

4   Working with emotions   56
Supervision as a space for emotional
   containment 56
Overwhelm 59
Disappointment 60
Anger 62
Shame 65
Anxiety 67
Grief 71
Summary 74

5   Working with relational dynamics   76
Personality, beliefs, and values 76
The use of self-disclosure 79
Counter-transference and parallel process 80
Transactional analysis 83
The problem is the problem not the person 86
Summary 87

6   Connecting to compassion   89
Defining compassion 89
Self-awareness 91
Emotional regulation 92
Anchor to core motivation 94
Consciously engage to develop
   acceptance, understanding and connection 95
Self-compassion and self-forgiveness 99
Summary 103

7   Supporting courage, grit, and resilience   105
Defining courage 106
Questions to connect courage 109
Grit 110
Resilience 112
Summary 114

8   **Strengthening holistic wellbeing**   116
    A holistic model of wellbeing 116
    *Supporting the parasympathetic nervous
        system 118*
    Building mental fitness 120
    Organisational culture 124
    Supervisor wellbeing 128
    Summary 129

Conclusion   131

Index   135

Figures

7.1   Process model of courage   108

Tables

8.1   Sphere well-being assessment (Weld, 2014)   117

Foreword

Whilst reading this book and wondering how to structure this foreword, the metaphors of digestion and nutrition came to mind. These particular metaphors arose from my musings on what the function of a foreword was exactly, and how I could write something that appropriately preceded the content of the book itself. It was at this point in my ruminations that the image of an appetiser came to mind – something to 'whet the appetite' in anticipation of the main meal. Psychotherapy often uses the language of nutrition, digestion, and metabolising processes to describe the emotional processes that we experience in our relationships with ourselves and each other. The cross-fertilisation of physiological and psychological processes is a generative one as it illustrates what is required for us to experience good physical and mental health. So, with this serendipitous inter-twining of my (seemingly) idiosyncratic reflections on reading this book, with the established psychotherapeutic practice of using nutritional metaphorical devices to understand human dynamics, let's tuck in.

Good supervision is like a nutritious meal that needs to be eaten slowly to appreciate all its flavours and ingredients. This book sets out a model of supervision, full of deep flavours and rich ingredients, that is both counter-cultural and paradoxical. Firstly, its attention to the process and dynamics of supervision runs counter to the culture of the managerial models of supervision that pervade the human service professions; and secondly, whilst it focuses on the therapeutic ingredients of supervision processes and relationships, it simultaneously firmly underlines that supervision is NOT therapy and a firm boundary must be held between these two distinctive types of activities. The meal, therefore, is an unusual one, not often on the menu for human service professionals, offering refreshing and critical perspectives, that draw on therapeutically-informed theoretical and practice-based knowledge. This luxurious mix of ingredients makes for a healthy, balanced diet.

Delving into the book we discover that each chapter is a meal in itself and requires careful attention in order to absorb and digest all the theoretical ideas, references, and case material that is on offer to the reader. Nicki brings to her writing a wealth of tastes and textures, drawing on well-informed theoretical understanding of therapeutic concepts, humanely illustrated with examples from her own supervision practice. As the reader–consumer – one feels confident that the 'chef' knows what they are creating and 'putting on the table'. And this confidence is enhanced by the openness of Nicki to her own vulnerabilities and ongoing learning.

> I like to bring misses, judgments, dilemmas, doubts, and emotional reactions to supervision. It is here I gain the greatest professional and personal learning which ultimately benefits those I am working with. As supervisees, we need to bring the mistakes, the successes, the moments of bewilderment and regret, emotional reactivity, and loss of regulation. We need to surface our unconscious bias, and our beliefs, values, attitudes and assumptions, and place them in the middle of the supervision space so we can critically examine them.
>
> (p. 15)

The book is a deeply reassuring one because of its honest engagement with the difficult task of supervision. As supervisors the challenge is always to be, not just double-edged, but triple-edged as we are required to hold in mind the vulnerable person requiring help, through holding the supervisee in mind, in turn through holding oneself as a supervisor in mind. Throughout the book there are constant reminders that one can only listen and respond to emotional difficulty and distress to the extent that, as a supervisor, you have been, and are being, listened to. Using the nutritional metaphor we can only feed and nourish others if we too are fed and nourished. In adopting such a transparent tone it offers a nourishing meal that feeds not just the body but also the soul. The whole person will feel better for engaging with these complex ideas that are set out so comprehensively and clearly.

Finally, it is imperative to acknowledge how cultural diversity is represented in the book, with its numerous references to Māori customs and the importance of first nation experiences for our understanding of human relations.

Cultural humility also embraces the concept of ako, drawn from Māori wisdom, which upholds reciprocity of learning from each other, where knowledge is socially constructed between both supervisor and supervisee.

(Hair & O'Donoghue, 2009, p. 58)

Writing from the context of the United Kingdom our need for cultural humility in human service practice is greater than ever. We need to ensure our dietary provision in supervision is inclusive and representative of the cultural diversity that characterises our global world.

So I heartedly recommend this book to you. Read it mindfully, digest it slowly, and experience being nourished and fed, in order to nourish and feed others.

Gillian Ruch
Professor of Social Work,
University of Sussex,
United Kingdom

Reference

Hair, H., & O'Donoghue, K. (2009). Culturally relevant, socially just social work supervision: Becoming visible through a social constructionist lens, *Journal of Ethnic & Cultural Diversity in Social Work, 18*(1–2), 70–88, DOI: 10.1080/15313200902874979.

Introduction

Worldwide issues such as climate change and the global pandemic, along with rising levels of stress, anxiety, and depression, are impacting individuals and communities. With limited formal mental health resources, many human service workers are finding themselves engaged in therapeutic work to support the psychological, physical, and emotional wellness of those they work with. Human service workers are also not personally immune to these increasing social complexities, often both working with these challenges and personally experiencing them.

Professional supervision is a key resource to help manage professional and personal responses (Carroll, 2014) especially when workers are providing therapeutic work to support complex emotional issues. This has become more evident and indeed critical, as we learn more about emotional labour, stress, distress, trauma, and indirect trauma from human service practice. We accept that we cannot walk into people's worlds without being touched by their stories and experiences, to not be, would indicate detachment to the point of being desensitised. Alternatively, to be overwhelmed by the people's experiences can also contribute to self protectively withdrawing from relational connection. This may result in under responsive practice evident in professional dangerousness, a phenomenon observed in child protection work where workers unwittingly collude with, maintain, or increase dangerous dynamics in families (Reder, Duncan & Gray, 1993, Morrison, 1990).

The western world tendency to over-label experiences as 'traumatic' invites the importance of making a distinction between the different forms of personal emotional responses workers may experience. 'Emotional labour' was first described by Hochschild in 1983, who developed this sociological concept based on research undertaken with flight attendants and debt collectors. She identified the labour

DOI: 10.4324/9781003359036-1

of having to suppress or induce emotion, often many times a day, and the resulting fatigue from this. This included the effort of having to produce an outward emotional state for another person, so 'surface acting' (Hochschild, 1983, p. 33), and for the worker to internally suppress what they might actually be feeling.

Miller and Sprang (2017) linked the concept of emotional labour to compassion fatigue observed in therapists, where the same effort of suppressing or inducing emotional responses may occur, namely when trying to maintain empathetic engagement. They noted this was more evident when working with behaviours that were challenging for the therapist, possibly even disliked by them. To remain in relationship with a person whose behaviour we find difficult or even abhorrent requires significant effort, and the management of our feelings to do this can be fatiguing.

Winter, Morrison, Cree, Ruch, Hadfield, and Halett (2019) expanded on the concept of emotional labour in their research with social workers in child protection. They noted that there can also be organisational expectations on how workers should respond emotionally. There can be covert and overt work cultures that induce workers to overly contain or suppress their emotions, and even deny feelings such as being scared or frightened. This was highlighted within the concept of the professional accommodation syndrome (Morrison, 1990) whereby organisational culture impedes and suppresses the worker's experience of the inherent anxiety found in child protection work.

Stress is registered through the mind in thoughts, feelings, and reactions, and experienced physiologically, often as strain or tension. Events that generate a stress or tension response can be episodic, so a time limited one-off event such as a workplace accident, or experienced frequently, such as working with unpredictable behaviour. Some short-term stress can be healthy and positive and can help increase alertness and focus, like getting ready for a new learning experience. Short-term stress helps us build our capacity for resiliency to manage in more challenging times.

There are also long-term or chronic stressful situations such as the emotional pressure of working in an organisational culture with persistent feelings of being undervalued, unseen, unaccepted, insignificant, insecure, or experiencing a lack of belonging, meaning, or autonomy (Wilson, 2018). Chronic stress might also be experienced from working with high levels of unpredictability such as clients having episodes of violent behaviour. We now know chronic stress can become toxic, especially impacting physical wellbeing, where it can cause inflammatory and autoimmune changes, namely through levels of increased cortisol. This can impact both physical and psychological health, contributing to burnout and poor staff retention. Supervision has a key role in supporting workers to be able to process and discharge chronic stress, so it does not have these consequences.

Distress indicates a partial or full overwhelming of coping capacity, and this may be linked to an event that disrupts a person's physical or psychological safety. It is these types of events or situations that can be considered traumatic, as they are more likely to contain confusing levels of sensory stimuli and cause difficulty in making sense of what is happening.

Acute traumatic events are usually time limited, so sudden overwhelming events that induce a physical or psychological threat to us or others (Levenson, 2017). They often happen quickly with little time to process or make sense of them, or can persist over a long period of time, essentially eroding our capacity to keep managing and coping. An example of this would be a natural disaster such as a major earthquake where impacts continue, such as aftershocks and unresolved damage to property. These types of experiences require time to be fully integrated and made sense of, and pre-existing vulnerabilities such as financial difficulties or multiple carer responsibilities can worsen the distress and stress from them (Adamson, 2018). Other situations such as accidents and a sudden threat to life such as a physical assault are also examples of acute traumatic events.

In response to these acute or prolonged overwhelming events, we can experience fear, helplessness, and an overwhelm of our normal coping mechanisms. This may persist for a few days or up to a month causing symptoms seen within Acute Stress Disorder which is indicated by physiological arousal, emotional distress, cognitive disturbance, withdrawal from usual activities, low mood, anxiety, disturbed sleep, and guilt. Opportunity to process these events and our reactions to them, along with increased access to social supports, can assist with the processing of the experience and restore coping.

Without this type of support and care, Post-Traumatic Stress Disorder (PTSD) can develop, characterised by persistent symptoms of arousal, intrusion, avoidance, and distress which can continue for years if not treated. PTSD is often more likely the result of exposure to prolonged traumatic events and being in close proximity to these. The condition was originally diagnosed and named in war veterans from the Vietnam wars, with an earlier term of 'shell shock' applied to veterans from the Great Wars. Although the term PTSD has replaced that of shell-shock, the older term remains useful in visualising a profound and often prolonged shock to the central nervous system.

Chronic trauma (or sometimes described as cumulative trauma) involves high levels of distress experienced frequently such as living with a lack of psychological and physical safety as experienced in family harm or countries affected by war. Chronic trauma becomes complex when secondary impacts occur in addition to the primary trauma. For example, a child living in family violence and neglect at home may struggle to form social relationships at school and then experience bullying. Chronic trauma in young children can cause developmental trauma observed through impacts on all aspects of brain development. It can also cause fundamental physiological changes with the physical stress response becoming permanently set in survival mode, impacting heart rate, endocrine and auto immune functionality.

Also stemming from relational traumatic events, Complex Post-Traumatic Stress Disorder (CPTSD) contains the symptomology of PTSD and also includes negative self-perception, low self-worth, and struggling to form or keep relationships. There is overall difficulty with emotional regulation, evidenced through anger and dissociative behaviours, along with physiological symptoms. CPTSD is typically caused by acute and chronic relational traumatic events, especially in childhood, but is also caused by violent adult relationships and being made to witness violent acts toward others.

We are also learning more about the impact of historical or multigenerational trauma, especially in the context of culture, such as ethnic and religious groups who experienced the devastation of genocide, slavery, and colonisation. The multiple impacts that persist to this day from these events contribute to layers of disadvantage with social, emotional, and physiological consequences for individuals and groups. It is not untypical in social service work to be working with an individual or family who presents with acute, chronic, complex, and historical multigenerational trauma.

In response to stress, distress, and trauma in service users or clients, general therapeutic work can be simply explained as the intentional restoring and strengthening of a person's emotional and psychological ability to manage not easily resolved and challenging life issues. A human service worker provides a safe relationship in which people can emotionally adapt and work through those life events. Events that have been overwhelming and disrupting of existing coping mechanisms, often reduce the person to a daily surviving, rather than living to their full potential, and a therapeutic relationship supports people to move beyond this. Harm that has occurred through a relationship is best healed through positive relational experiences, and in human service work we provide the supportive connection for recovery to occur within.

While workers themselves can directly experience acute and chronic traumatic events, as well as having histories of chronic, complex, and multigenerational trauma, we now understand that exposure to the traumatic stories and experiences of those they work with can also cause secondary or indirect trauma impacts for them. Vicarious traumatisation, secondary traumatic stress, and compassion fatigue are the three main forms of indirect trauma experienced through indirect exposure to experiences of suffering and harm.

Initially observed in psychotherapists, vicarious traumatisation can be described as 'negative transformation of the therapist's inner experience' and 'close empathetic engagement' with clients who have experienced trauma (Saakvitne, 2002, p. 446). Changes may occur in beliefs, values, sense of efficacy, and overall self-perception and identity. There can be persistent feelings of hopelessness and helplessness through being in daily contact with the distress and suffering of others. Vicarious traumatisation tends to happen over time, and can be indicated by loss of hope, increased helplessness, fear, and self-doubt about one's role and purpose.

Secondary Traumatic Stress (STS) can have a much more rapid onset than vicarious traumatisation, usually through secondary or indirect exposure to traumatic material, such as hearing the details of this, or seeing the impact of it. This, in turn, causes longer term post-traumatic stress type symptoms in workers including: having difficulty managing emotional responses such as experiencing distress and being easily upset, avoidance such as withdrawing from client situations too early, intrusion such as having disrupted sleep, and increased arousal such as having a heightened reaction to a situation where the intensity of response is not warranted. Kellogg (2021) also notes that STS symptoms can also mirror those of Acute Stress Disorder, while proposing that STS is 'an intrusive state of psychological tension resulting from witnessing the emotional or physical suffering of another as part of a professional helping relationship' (p. 166).

While not limited solely to exposure of trauma and suffering, compassion fatigue becomes evident through decreased compassion and empathy, a need to relationally and socially withdraw, increased reactivity, sleep disturbance, physical unwellness, and avoidance of emotionally demanding situations. As mentioned, compassion fatigue is linked to the concept of emotional labour (Miller & Sprang

2017) where workers are engaged in high levels of effort to induce or suppress their emotional responses in order to generate an empathetic response.

Miller and Sprang (2017) identify this is especially evident if the worker is experiencing countertransference from their own personal histories of trauma and who then seek to self-protectively withdraw from relational engagement. Singer, Cummings, Boekankamp, Hisaka, Benuto (2020) in their research with victim support advocates also note a high correlation between workers with their own relational trauma histories and a vulnerability to compassion fatigue and burnout. Compassion fatigue is more likely to arise when there is failure to distinguish between empathy and countertransference (Miller & Sprang, 2017, p. 155). Workers who have high levels of empathy can join with the emotional experiences of the client and invest significant amounts of their own emotional energy. When coupled with unconscious countertransference, as an underlying trigger, this can lead to fatigue.

This invites a rethink of the term 'compassion fatigue' when perhaps what is occurring is 'empathy fatigue'. Compassion, when applied intentionally and effectively, contributes to compassion satisfaction – the sense of increased accomplishment, positivity, motivation, and fulfilling connection in our work with others rather than fatigue (Singer, Cummings, Boekankamp, Hisaka & Benuto, 2020). It can sustain workers and be an enriching process rather than one that is draining or exhausting. The application of compassion is discussed further in Chapter 6 as a preventative measure to indirect trauma.

Vicarious trauma, secondary traumatic stress, and compassion fatigue are not inevitable for social service workers but do require supervisors to be able to notice, recognise and respond to these impacts. Left unattended, indirect trauma impacts can contribute to other workplace stressors such as overwhelming workloads and an unsupportive organisational culture. These wider system impacts can lead to burnout where workers become depleted, cynical, emotionally and physically exhausted, negative about their work, dissatisfied, and effectively withdraw from their work and workplace (Singer, Cummings, Boekankamp, Hisaka & Benuto, 2020).

There may also be times when a worker experiences both their own direct traumatic response to an event, along with secondary exposure through working with others who experienced that event, so a dual response. This was evident in hospital workers who both experienced the Aotearoa New Zealand Canterbury earthquakes then worked with survivors of these, and in the health workforce managing the impacts of COVID-19 pandemic.

The emotional impacts of human service work in our current global environment have elevated the need for supervision to provide an intentional therapeutic function. If workers are not well and lacking the opportunity to integrate stress, distress, trauma, emotional labour, and indirect trauma impacts, there are serious consequences for professional practice, which, in turn, can cause workers further distress. Articulating a therapeutic function of professional supervision extends the traditional restorative function (Proctor, 1987) and supportive function (Kadussin & Harkness, 2014) to intentionally acknowledge and respond to the emotional impacts of human service work along with the supporting of the development of grit and resilience to manage these in the future.

There can be discomfort about providing a therapeutic function in supervision which will be explored in the first chapter beginning with defining different types of supervision. In Chapter 2, attuning and attending are discussed among a range of ways to support a relational foundation in which the therapeutic function can be enacted. In Chapter 3 the power of developing a coherent narrative is explored as a way of inviting integration of traumatic experiences. The importance of emotions as critical sources of information and ways to help with regulation of these is examined in Chapter 4. Exploring emotions also helps make sense of the impacts from relational dynamics which are discussed in Chapter 5. Two core components of therapeutic work, compassion, and courage are applied to the supervision experience in Chapters 6 and 7, along with the concepts of grit and resilience. Finally, supporting holistic wellbeing and optimising mental health is discussed in Chapter 8.

Poor delivery of key professional support systems such as professional supervision leaves workers alternatively exposed, displaced emotionally, and struggling to hold the emotional impacts of human service work. Ultimately supervision is a source of professional development to support quality service delivery often to people experiencing a range of vulnerabilities and impacts. As supervisors we have a responsibility that those delivering these services are safe and well, and able to bring the very best of themselves to their work. Hawkins and Shohet (2012) comment that 'supervision is not just about preventing stress and burnout however but enables supervisees to continually learn and flourish so they spend more time working at their best' (p. 6). The time has come to articulate the therapeutic function in supervision to attend to the emotional impacts of human service work so workers can indeed be at their best.

References

Adamson, C. (2018). Trauma-informed supervision in the disaster context. *The Clinical Supervisor, 37*(1), 221–240. DOI: 10.1080/07325223. 2018.1426511.

Carroll, M. (2014). *Effective supervision for the helping professions.* London: Sage Publications.

Hawkins, P., & Shohet, R. (2012). *Ebook: Supervision in the helping professions.* Berkshire: McGraw-Hill Education.

Hochschild, A. R. (1983). *The Managed Heart.* Berkeley: University of California Press.

Kadusshin, A., & Harkness, D. (2014). *Supervision in social work.* New York: Columbia University Press.

Kellogg, M. (2021). Secondary traumatic stress in nursing. *Advances in Nursing Science, 44*(2), 157–170. DOI: 10.1097/ANS.0000000000000338.

Levenson, J. (2017). Trauma-informed social work practice. *Social Work, 62*(2), 105–113.

Miller, B., & Sprang, G. (2017). A components-based practice and supervision model for reducing compassion fatigue by affecting clinician experience. *Traumatology, 23*(2), 153–164. DOI: 10.1037/trm0000058.

Morrison, T. (1990). The emotional effects of child protection work on the worker. *Practice, 4*(4), 253–271. DOI: 10.1080/09503159008416902.

Proctor, B. (1987). Supervision: A co-operative exercise in accountability. In M. Marken, & M. Payne (Eds.), *Enabling and ensuring: Supervision in practice* (pp. 21–34). Leister: National Youth Bureau and the Council for Education and Training in Youth and Community Work.

Reder, P., Duncan, S., & Gray, M. (1993). *Beyond blame.* London. Routledge.

Saakvitne, K. W. (2002). Shared trauma: The therapist's increased vulnerability. *Psychoanalytic Dialogues, 12*, 443–449. DOI: 10.1080/10481881209348678.

Singer, J., Cummings, C., Boekankamp, D., Hisaka, R., & Benuto, L. T. (2020). Compassion satisfaction, compassion fatigue, and burnout: A replication study with victim advocates. *Journal of Social Service Research, 46*(3), 313–319. DOI: 10.1080/01488376.2018.1561595.

Wilson, B. (2018). How to fix the exhausted brain. TED Talk. https://www.youtube.com/watch?v=XOU2ubWkoPw.

Winter, K., Morrison, F., Cree, V., Ruch, G., Hadfield, M., & Hallet, S. (2019). Emotional labour in social workers' encounters with children and their families. *British Journal of Social Work, 49*(1), 217–233. ISSN 0045-3102.

1   Defining the therapeutic function of supervision

Engaging a therapeutic function in supervision can create anxiety for some supervisors who worry they may cross into the territory of therapy and confuse their role of supervisor with that of a therapist. This boundary needs to be defined so supervisors and supervisees both maintain role clarity, and the emotional impacts of the work are safely able to be integrated and managed. It begins with clearly defining different types of supervision, the role of the supervisor in professional supervision, and the functions of supervision. By making a distinction between providing a therapeutic function, and engaging in therapy, supervisors will have more confidence to work with the emotional impacts of social service work on supervisees.

Types of supervision

Supervision exists in a variety of ways that support organisational safety and staff retention and promote practice excellence and professional development (Karvinen-Niinikoski, Beddoe, Ruch & Tsui, 2019). It may be mandated by professions to meet professional registration requirements and/or required by an organisation and underpinned by a supervision policy. It can be provided internally or externally, and sometimes a combination of the two.

Within the context of individual supervision, the three main forms are line management, clinical, and professional. Supervision can also occur in a group context where several practitioners might meet with an independent facilitator, or with others in a peer-based arrangement. Group and peer supervision should not replace individual supervision but can provide an additional means of support and learning.

In larger organisations, particularly those providing internal supervision, there can be a blurring of line management supervision, clinical supervision, and professional supervision, due to a possible lack of

DOI: 10.4324/9781003359036-2

clarity and understanding. It is important that the different types of individual supervision can be clearly identified and articulated within organisations and understood by management and practitioners.

Line management or administrative supervision provides oversight and accountability of an organisation's outcomes, activities, and standards to ensure the provision of a quality service. This includes effective and appropriate implementation of agency policies and procedures and compliance with these. It helps provide staff with the resources and systems to manage them in their roles. Tasks of line management supervision include delegation and workload management, performance appraisal, duty of care, support, and other people-management processes. The person providing the supervision may be in a team leader or managerial role, and therefore has authority in the relationship with the worker. They will largely determine the agenda of the session, predicted by organisational requirements.

When I worked in a hospital setting as a professional leader of social work, I had line management supervision with the operations manager of allied health. In this supervision we discussed areas such as my work plan and aligning this to wider organisational direction and expectation.

Clinical supervision has a focus on clinical practice development in a key area or modality of practice. It assists with developing skills, techniques, meeting practice standards, and provides clinical direction and support. This might include developing greater cultural responsiveness when working with a cultural group different to one's own. The overall focus is to enhance clinical expertise, competence, and confidence. It can be provided by someone from a different professional discipline to the worker who has expertise in that field of practice or by a practice leader within the workers own profession. Clinical supervision is critical to the development of practice skill and competency, and can have an intern aspect to it, where coaching and mentoring helps the development of key skills and knowledge. It therefore can have a 'student/expert' orientation, with a teaching focus (Davys & Beddoe, 2020) which may also carry an assessment and performance requirement.

When I worked as a national social work advisor in a non-government organisation, I provided clinical supervision to social workers experiencing challenge or difficulty in their clinical practice with a child or family. An example might be a family where significant care and protection issues were apparent and the worker was seeking supervision on best practice to address these. My focus was more on the details of the child and family situation, exploring what had been tried and providing clinical guidance as to where to next. I did not necessarily have an existing relationship with the worker, and was solely working with the clinical challenge they were experiencing.

Professional supervision provides a protected time for critical in-depth discovery and reflection that supports the integration of experience into professional and personal learning. Ingham comments that reflection involves "thinking about and reviewing one's practice and considering the context, knowledge, inter/intra personal dynamics and outcomes at play, and considering how this learning may impact on current understanding and future practice" (Ingham, 2015, cited in Ingham, 2021, p. 464). Carroll (2014) states that "co-created reflective learning is the heart of supervision" (p. 26).

This includes exploring roles and relationships, the worker's practice, and personal and contextual factors that impact the work as described within the Seven Eyed model of supervision developed by Hawkins. In this model, the supervisee is invited to reflect relationally and systemically on (1) what is happening for the client, (2) the interventions they have undertaken in relation to the client, (3) the relationship between themselves and the client including any issues of transference, and (4) the internal processes at play for the supervisee in relation to the client including examining possible countertransference. The supervisor reflects on (5) the supervisory relationship including any parallel process they might be experiencing in relation to the supervisee, (6) their here and now responses to the supervisee and what has been shared about the client, and (7) both examine the wider systems in which this relational work between the client, supervisee, and supervisor is taking place (Hawkins & Shohet, 2012, pp. 87–88).

In professional supervision it is the supervisee who decides on the agenda for a session, indicative that this is their time to explore and reflect. Paulin (2010) notes that supervision is "supervisee-led but supervisor facilitated" (p. 107). It is a professional contracted activity, focused on ensuring professional accountability, learning and reflection, in which practitioners are engaged throughout the duration of their careers regardless of experience or qualification (Davys and Beddoe, 2020, pp. 22, 36). Ultimately professional supervision supports quality service delivery through focused support and critique, and assists the worker to achieve and sustain a high quality of professional, and also, personal development (Davys and Beddoe, 2020).

Professional supervision is dependent on a safe, trusting relationship which Webber-Dreadon (2020) highlights in her challenge of the term 'supervision' instead describing the concept of Kaitiakitanga.

Her definition of Kaitiakitanga emphasises an action to support, uphold and maintain responsible, trustworthy engagement between the supervisor and the supervisee (Webber-Dreadon, 2020). She identifies Kaitiakitanga to be a "socially, heartfelt and humanist approach" with concern firstly for those people that a supervisee is working with including their physical, emotional needs and spiritual needs, their welfare, their values, and their dignity (Webber-Dreadon, 2020, p. 70). The role of the supervisor is to watch over, to care for, guide, nurture and protect those who the supervisee is working for and with, as well as the supervisee themselves (Webber-Dreadon, 2020).

In reviewing supervision articles and research, O'Donoghue notes that supervisees identify the key purpose of professional supervision as being to develop "knowledge and skills, as well as the provision of emotional support" (O'Donoghue, 2021, p. 643). Professional supervision attends to the "emotional content of the work" (Miller, 2018) and is therefore an ideal space to address the impacts of emotional labour, stress, distress, trauma, and indirect trauma impacts. It provides a place to temporarily reflect and restore, to think and wonder out loud, to unpack and test assumptions, gather evidence, and test the validity of one's thinking. It is the worker's time to explore, gain clarity, and process the junction of their internal and external worlds. The supervisor is the facilitator of this, while also being open to learning and providing challenge and being receptive to receiving this.

While some crossover of function may occur between clinical and professional supervision, in my observation, the main difficulty emerges when line management roles exist in professional supervision, namely through the supervisor having organisational authority over the worker. This creates the dynamic of 'guarding' (Herkt & Hocking, 2007) where workers, aware of the power disparity and imbalance of authority, protect what they share in supervision due to a worry of how this information might be used. They therefore consciously or unconsciously guard their practice by using cognitive avoidance strategies or physically avoiding supervision by not making time for it (Herkt & Hocking, 2007, p. 28).

Naming difficulty around coping with emotional impacts of the work or stress in a guarded session is unlikely to occur, and if this is the only form of supervision available to the worker, then their emotional experiences will not be adequately identified, expressed, or processed. Learning and development is likely to be stunted, confined to complying with organisational expectations, and runs the risk of 'cloning' (Carroll, 2014) clinical practice. If there is also a significant power differential due to the supervisor holding managerial responsibilities, the supervisee's heightened awareness of this may impair critical reflection, insight, and learning. It is therefore essential for supervisors to be clear about the type of supervision they are providing, their role within this, and any organisational power they hold.

Bond and Holland (2011) provide a useful criteria checklist for nurses when choosing a professional supervisor that includes:

- Skills in enabling in-depth reflection
- Relevant professional background
- No line management responsibility
- Some understanding of your role
- Not working closely with you
- Able to keep confidentiality
- No personal relationship

(Bond & Holland, 2011, p. 97)

Within this criterion are clear indicators about what professional supervision is and is not, such as line management, and it also highlights potential conflicts of interest such as supervision with a friend or relative. Hawkins and Shohet (2012) summarise supervision as supporting development through an educator function, providing support, and overseeing the quality of the supervisee's work with clients. They do however note that supervisors can sometimes retreat to just one of these roles, becoming facilitators of case consults, becoming quasi counsellors, or delivering a managerial checklist (Hawkins & Shohet, 2012, p. 5).

Interdisciplinary supervision

Professional supervision can be provided across and between different professional disciplines. It is preferable in the early stages of career to receive professional supervision from within one's own professional discipline to support the development of professional identity. More experienced practitioners may receive professional supervision in an interdisciplinary supervisory relationship. Here the supervisor is not necessarily from the same professional occupation, including holding different training and qualification. The supervisee will therefore need to have an identified person they can receive specific clinical guidance from.

For example, I am not qualified to provide clinical direction to medical doctors I provide professional supervision to, they receive this from other medical doctors and consultants. However, I can support their practice by enabling them to engage in broader reflection which will assist them with integration of their experiences into learning and knowledge. I have developed this book from my interdisciplinary supervisory practice encompassing the professions of social work, counselling, nursing, law, medicine, management, tertiary education, and police.

My supervisory practice is influenced by my professional identity as a social worker, something I openly acknowledge to possible new supervisees. Other supervisors might have a professional background in allied health or psychology which informs their supervisory practice. In an external interdisciplinary model of supervision, the supervisee makes a choice if they wish to have supervision from someone with the same professional qualification or one that is different. While professional supervision is a profession in its own right (Carroll, 2014), and one that contains generic reflective processes, the influence of the supervisor's professional background will likely be evident. The lens that has shaped our professional worldview will continue to be present in the practice of supervision.

Key principles of interprofessional supervision include:

1 Providing an objective, safe critically reflective space to explore and analyse a person's role, practice, and self.
2 Acknowledging diversity and difference, showing curiosity and interest in this, and linking through the common ground of social service/people work.
3 Displaying and applying relational qualities of trust, respect, interest, curiosity, appreciation, and warmth.
4 Demonstrating a commitment to partnering for high quality service delivery, safe practice, and worker wellbeing.
5 That direct clinical guidance and accountability must be present for the supervisee typically within their organisation.

(Adapted, Davys, Fouché & Beddoe, 2021)

Interdisciplinary supervision brings an advantage of a cross fertilisation of knowledge, where both supervisor and supervisee learn about the other's professions. Due to having to ask into areas not known due to the difference in profession, this itself invites greater reflection through the process of explaining. Davys and Beddoe (2020) comment that this level of exploration and explanation "can bring forth new ideas and challenge practice which has previously been accepted without question" (p. 68). There can be an exchange of ideas which support the notion of reciprocity of learning, and this can be mutually satisfying. This helps increase understanding, appreciation, and respect for other professions (O'Donoghue, 2021).

Roles in professional supervision

To provide professional supervision, the supervisor must be credible in their own profession with at least three years of professional experience, and must have undertaken training in professional supervision, recognising that it is a unique role with its own set of skills. The supervisor engages in a partnership with the supervisee that evidences mutual respect, honesty, and trust, with a clear intention and commitment to support professional and personal development. The supervisor's role is to support role clarity and competence, and to contribute to the supervisee's practice wisdom, self-knowledge, and self-awareness through enabling critical reflection and encouraging further education.

The supervisee's role requires active involvement in both the session and supervisory relationship. Claiming the time as their own, preparing, and participating fully mean that a worker is not simply 'receiving supervision' but being a co-creator in the dynamic process of building and sharing knowledge. While the supervisor acts as a facilitator to integrate experience into learning, this is wholly dependent on what the supervisee brings to supervision and how responsive they are to questions, observations, and challenge.

I like to bring misses, judgements, dilemmas, doubts, and emotional reactions to supervision. It is here I gain the greatest professional and personal learning which ultimately benefits those I am working with. As supervisees, we need to bring the mistakes, the successes, the moments of bewilderment and regret, emotional reactivity, and loss of regulation. We need to surface our unconscious bias, and our beliefs, values, attitudes, and assumptions and place them in the middle of the supervision space so we can critically examine them.

Critical reflection involves consideration of the influences in the wider socio-political context, organisational culture, and environment including surfacing and examining power, dominant discourses, and issues of inequity especially in social work. The deconstruction of these wider influences contributes to the supervisee understanding and potentially reconstructing these to evidence "changes in awareness and action" (Rankine, 2021, p. 347). Critical reflection looks both "inward and outwards" (Fook, 2015, p. 443) involving metacognition (thinking about ones thinking) and the examination of assumptions and beliefs. Turney and Ruch (2018) comment that reflective spaces enable people to "get beneath the surface" and "think around the edges" (p. 129). It is supported by the application of skilled questioning to facilitate analysis (Rankine, 2021) with the intention to re-develop or strengthen personal and professional practice thinking and learning.

Dedicating time and space to critically reflect is essential in roles which are highly emotionally demanding. A number of authors including Ruch (2005), Casement (1985) and Ferguson (2018) comment on how workers limit reflection in order to emotionally defend and contain. Not having space to reflect and process these emotional responses, can leave workers in a state of persistent emotional defending which interrupts cognitive processing to support decision making. In my experience, these workers can present as disconnected from clients, or in a state of emotional disintegration evidenced by overwhelm and poor decision making.

To provide a safe (and brave) reflective space, the supervisor and supervisee needs to be able to create a supportive relational environment that encourages the sharing and exploration of experience. The Kaitiakitanga approach supports the emphasis on relationship with the Māori principles of Kōrero Awhi (positive communication), Tika (best practice), Manaakitanga (respect and compassion), Kaupapa (having a collective vision), Pūmanawa (natural talents), Whakamana (empowerment), Whānau (a sense of belonging), Mā Tauranga (knowledge and wisdom), and Mauri ora (wellbeing) which enable trust and mirror ideal practice with people (Webber-Dreadon, 2020, p. 75).

For trust to be present, the supervisor must demonstrate warmth, care, honesty, interest, and be reliable with a clear commitment to the supervision relationship. To support critical thinking, it helps if a supervisor is a creative and critical thinker themselves, with an ability to be curious which is reflected in the questions they ask and techniques they apply. The supervisor respects the autonomy of the supervisee and is committed to being a shared solution finder with them.

It is essential that the supervisor does not create an over reliance or dependency upon themselves to find answers, instead ensuring that the supervisee builds their own solutions and takes responsibility for the actions they take. While the supervisor is responsible for any advice or suggestions they might make, it is ultimately the supervisee who chooses to act (or not) on these and is responsible for their own actions. Key skills a supervisor can bring to support the therapeutic function will be discussed further in the next chapter.

Overall, the supervisor is the facilitator of a reflective process that involves increasing self-awareness, critical analysis, and learning that contributes to new perspectives (Thorpe, 2004) and the development of knowledge. They navigate between the domains of professional role, practice, and self, and contribute observations and questions to assist in the supervisee's integration of experience into professional and personal wisdom. It is a role that carries significant responsibility as the supervisor must be vigilant to unsafe practice including possible impacts of an imbalance in the wellbeing of the supervisee. The supervisor must remain alert to practice that is harmful or detrimental to clients, including being aware of potential professional dangerousness.

The supervisee commits to being an active participant in the reflective learning process and it is through what they bring to explore and integrate that provides the content of the session. They remain responsible for their practice decisions and take responsibility for their own development of knowledge along with attendance to wellbeing and safety. It is essential that a supervisee recognise if their supervision is no longer meeting their needs and take steps to address this through requesting what they need or ending the supervisory relationship. They must be able to challenge the supervisor if they perceive unsafe or unwell practice, just as the supervisor needs to supportively challenge them. Professional supervision can be a rare, protected space for reflection in often very busy work environments. It is essential that it is effective in fulfilling the overall focus of professional development to support service users.

External professional supervision therefore evidences partnership, not only with the supervisee, but also with the organisation and the wider service the supervisee works for. A clear contract is essential to outline the responsibilities of all parties engaged in the supervision provision, including what steps will be taken if the supervisor remains concerned about potentially harmful or impacted practice. This should include the provision for the external supervisor to raise any concerns they have about the organisation if they see this impacting negatively on workers' practice and wellbeing. There needs to be transparent acknowledgement in external supervision that the supervisor is typically paid by the organisation which signals a responsibility to the clients that the agency works with and for.

I liken this to the supervisor having a clear focus on the worker practice and wellbeing, while ultimately looking past them to see how this affects and impacts those they are engaged with. Therefore, a degree of monitoring is always operating, meaning that while a collaborative working partnership is strived for, power in the supervisory relationship is tipped in the direction of the supervisor. However, a supervisee should feel able to also signal concern about a supervisor's practice and wellbeing if this is warranted. It is therefore essential supervisors are also receiving their own professional supervision and are able to reflect on their supervision practice.

The supervisory space is therefore one of positive regard and a commitment to the co-development of knowledge, so learning with and learning from each other which uphold the knowledge and dignity of the supervisee and those they work with. Shohet (2011), quoting Carroll comments: "Supervision is an exciting and passionate journey in learning from experience and that learning journey, like all journeys, is filled with insights, self-awareness, challenges and surprises. Supervisors are heroes of learning" (p. 13).

The functions of professional supervision

Over the years, key functions of professional supervision have been described in a variety of ways, including by authors such as Proctor (1987), Morrison (1993, 2001), and Kadusshin and Harkness (2014). Along with educative and administrative functions, Kadusshin and Harkness (2014) discuss the supportive function of supervision, identifying this as improving and sustaining morale and job satisfaction (p. 9) with the intention of being able to offer clients an effective service. They note this attends to the inherent stresses in social service work that stem from the client relationship, supervision relationship, organisation demands, and community attitudes. In their work they identify the supportive function as providing relief, restoration, comfort and replenishment, along with inspiring and increasing job satisfaction (p. 162). This assists with the prevention of burnout and increased job satisfaction.

Along with a support function, Morrison (1993), draws on the work of Richards and Payne (1990) and also Proctor (1987) and adds management, education, and mediation functions, noting as other authors do, that exclusive focus on just one function reduces the overall effectiveness of supervision. When examining the support function, Morrison notes this includes examining the impact of the work on the supervisee as a person, and creating a space for feelings to be explored. The support function is seen to 'monitor the overall health and emotional functioning of the worker especially with regard the effects of stress' (p. 22). Morrison also notes that within this function is when a supervisor might advise a supervisee to seek external counselling.

Beddoe and Davys (2016) argue that support, rather than a function of supervision, is an "essential component of effective supervision" (p. 72), making it a required condition of supervision. This contributes to worker safety within the supervisory relationship, allowing for the exploration of practice and expression of vulnerability. Differentiating between a 'condition' and a 'function' of supervision would position a function as requiring purposeful and deliberate application with a specific focus or goal in mind.

Proctor (1987) provides description of three main functions of professional supervision as being normative, formative, and restorative. The addition of thinking from authors such as Davys and Beddoe (2020), drawing on the work of Hughes and Pengelly (1997), help position these three functions as the development of the professional, development of the worker's practice, and support of the practitioner, all of which contribute to service delivery (p. 35).

The normative function therefore supports reflection and development of ways and resources to enhance professional role, identity, responsibilities and performance. Focusing on this function helps facilitate the development of a strong professional identity and aligns this to understanding of and accountability to professional and organisational practice standards, ethics, governance frameworks, guidelines, and requirements. Reflection here supports understanding of a supervisee's role, that of others, and how to best manage relationships within immediate and wider teams or settings.

The formative function encourages reflection on knowledge and skills applied in practice with the intention of developing these, and helps the worker express, explore, and develop their practice. It builds and contributes to practice competence by facilitating critical reflection, and may include education and information that supports this. Exploration of practice situations include exploring ethical dilemmas and complex decision making including the need for courageous conversations.

Linking to the supportive function, the restorative function assists with ways to identify and plan strategies to support worker wellbeing. This can also include personal events outside of the professional workplace that have implications and impacts on a person's ability to work. There may also be times when workplace and practice events trigger personal issues for a worker, requiring support to process and then develop strategies to best manage these, including the possibility of accessing counselling or therapy support.

All three functions contribute to the overall intention of supporting a worker to undertake their professional duties with clarity and competence. One supervision session can involve all three functions, essentially strengthening how someone is doing in their role, their work, and how they are doing in themselves. Ultimately the functions support safe practice and professional growth that upholds quality service delivery for those the worker is engaged with.

I have expanded the traditional supportive and restorative functions of professional supervision to include a therapeutic function. I define this as intentionally attending to the emotional impacts of human service work to enable the integration of the experience and increasing self-awareness, self-knowledge, and emotional management skills. This in turn increases emotional capacity and ultimately contributes to the development of professional and personal grit and resilience. Impacts such as stress, distress, emotional labour, trauma, and indirect trauma require more than simply support. The intensity of experience should be matched by an appropriate level of response. The therapeutic function also provides for the consideration of personal and contextual factors which may impact professional practice.

The therapeutic and therapy boundary

Throughout the literature, the concern that supervision does not cross the boundary into therapy or counselling persists. Knapman and Morrison (1998) note that the support function is "not therapy or counselling but does recognise the role that feelings and emotions play in the caring work" (p. 10). Itzhaky and Itzhaky (1996) comment that the continued emphasis on making this distinction between supervision and therapy highlights the sensitivity to and challenge in holding the line between the two (p. 78). Hawkins and McMahon (2020) make reference to interviews with supervisors who referred to the dilemma of addressing person issues in supervision and their discomfort with this (p. 57).

The challenge of this boundary is most explicit in the fields of counselling and psychotherapy where a therapist moves into the role of being a supervisor. Page and Wosket (2015) take time to consider the differences between counselling and psychotherapy to that of supervision. They note that a therapy relationship holds a client emotionally with attention given to the dynamics of transference which may include regressed behaviour from the client. In comparison they recognise that supervision provides a container for the demands of counselling or therapy work, and has expectations that the relationship remains in an 'adult to adult' transaction. They also emphasise that in supervision, responsibility to the client may claim precedence to that of the supervisee, requiring supervisors to hold a greater use of authority (pp. 19, 20). They note that supervision is less emotionally demanding than therapy, however there are times where emotional and psychological issues of the supervisee do need attention drawn to them.

Page and Wosket (2015) comment that it is indeed necessary (and legitimate) to engage in a degree of therapeutic work with the supervisee (p. 24) however this must be related back to how it will serve the client. They bring attention to the need for a counsellor or therapist taking on the role of a supervisor, to have developed an understanding of models of supervision. They are then guided by an explicit focus on how the supervision they provide enables the counsellor or therapist to be of ultimate benefit to the client. This encapsulates the distinction between one's professional role, and being in the role as a supervisor. For myself, this requires me to differentiate my roles of being a social worker and being a supervisor, and the same question must be asked of anyone who makes the shift into the role of a supervisor from an existing professional base.

The goals of supervision and therapy are markedly different. Supervision holds the goal of contributing to and ensuring high quality service delivery through the enhancement of professional development. Itzhaky and Itzhaky (1996) notes that within the supervisory context there are three key people – the supervisee, the supervisor, and the client. This is not the case in a therapy context where there is only the therapist and the client. The functions of supervision are intended to contribute to the overarching aim of professional development that ultimately supports the client. When a supervisor is applying the therapeutic function of supervision, they should be asking themselves the question of 'How, in applying this function, will it support the clients that the supervisee is working with?'

The interchangeable use of the terms 'therapeutic' and 'therapy' in the previous century have likely exacerbated the worry between applying an intentional therapeutic function in supervision. With the emergence of a more articulated description of wellbeing and activities to support this, the distinction between therapy and therapeutic has become clearer.

Broadly defined, the term therapeutic encompasses a range of activities that contribute to wellbeing and help alleviate stress and strain. They might include undertaking actions that promote emotional coping and are restorative with an added dimension of increasing personal self-awareness and skills in emotional management. Engaging in therapeutic activities does not require a therapist as a person can do these on their own or with others. Engaging in a therapeutic activity is usually indicated by symptoms of emotional stress or distress, and a need to alleviate and build capacity to better address these in the future.

Unease around applying the therapeutic function of supervision may exist for supervisors who link the traditional connation of 'healing' found in the Greek word 'therapeutikos' from which therapeutic is derived. Healing likely conjures images of hands-on physical treatments or interventions which supervisors would be well advised to not engage in! However 'therapeutikos' can also mean 'attending' or 'restoring' and these concepts sit well within the supervisory space. In the next chapter we will see that attuned attending is a core component to be able to provide the therapeutic function of supervision. The notion of restorative is already an accepted function of supervision in application to supervisee wellbeing.

Therapy involves a specific psychodynamic, cognitive, or behavioural treatment or intervention to support often persistent emotional, psychological, or relational difficulties. This treatment is delivered by a trained professional in that modality. The therapist establishes a set of goals with the client to address these personal difficulties. Therapy, with its focus on personal growth, requires significant emotional disclosure and the relationship between therapist and client is itself a core source of information and is fundamental to the process of therapy, for example, in the area of transference.

I am suggesting that the supervisor, at times, enact a therapeutic function (just like the normative, educative, or formative functions) to attend to emotional impacts of the work, which is not about stepping into the role of a therapist. I had an example of this when a supervisee contacted me for an urgent supervision session. They had identified that they had become significantly distressed about a child neglect situation and were observing intrusive thoughts and images associated with this. On hearing of their distress I decided to apply the therapeutic function of supervision, so intentionally supporting the telling of the experience and exploration of their emotional response to help build a coherent narrative around what had occurred for them. Acknowledging I was applying the therapeutic function of supervision gave me permission to undertake a deep exploration of their emotional response to help them make sense of how they responded, deepen insight into their reaction, and begin to integrate the experience.

I spent about 40 minutes providing the therapeutic function of supervision, then began to move to the formative and normative functions, so exploring their practice and their role. My focus here was to help my supervisee re-engage with the family as their distress had caused them to withdraw, leaving the children vulnerable. Here we applied emotional knowledge gained from their reaction to the situation, and unpacked their thinking about their initial practice decision and their role and responsibilities within their service. We concluded the session with me applying scaling questions about the distress and they were able to name a reduction in this. We then discussed some simple self-care restorative activities for the evening ahead. At the end of the session they named relief from the distress and we had identified steps moving forward with the family that incorporated the key responsibilities of their role. The next day they contacted me to say that the emotional distress had gone and they were able to step back into engagement with the family.

The therapeutic function of supervision helps people to emotionally discharge what is front and centre, particularly in processing overt signs of emotional labour, stress, distress, trauma and indirect trauma. When these are present, a supervisor can intentionally apply the therapeutic function of supervision and will apply the other functions of supervision once the emotional impacts have been addressed.

Schamess (2006) positions that supervision is not therapy, but supervision sensitively offered does support personal change as well as professional development. He notes that "helpful supervision is intrinsically, continuously therapeutic" (p. 433). Beinart and Clohessy (2017) comment that "Although there is no evidence that good therapists always make good supervisors, there is some evidence to suggest that good supervisors use therapeutic qualities in supervision" (p. 31).

I find the therapeutic function of supervision is supported by my social work skills, especially the skill of supportive counselling if a supervisee is experiencing distress. Supportive counselling is the provision of emotional support, intended to normalise reactions, provide for the safe expression of what is happening, bring comfort, catharsis, clarity, perspective and guidance (Tripathi, 2005). It helps people to express emotions, process an event, and connect to their ways of coping. Very simply, it is the provision of a human presence in times of difficulty. While drawing on my social work skills, I recognise supervision is in itself, is its own unique practice, and the supervisee is not a social work client.

If known and relevant, the supervisor might occasionally make a connection to early life experiences of the supervisee but does not unpack these in a form of personal therapy. Just as I do not need to know every detail of a client situation but enough to have a context through which I can connect to the worker' s experience, it helps to have some personal understanding of each supervisee. Hawkins and McMahon (2020) comment that "Good supervision inevitably focusses some of its attention on the personal dynamics of supervisees, as working in the helping professions can restimulate personal feelings of distress, anger or anxiety" (p. 57). This recognition and understanding of the person beyond their professional role supports rapport, trust, relational warmth, and understanding.

An example of this was a supervisee who named they experienced serious abuse and violence in their childhood. I did not need to know the details of this, nor seek these, but being made aware of it helped me be mindful of possible vulnerabilities for them from a developmental trauma perspective. My supervisee generally functioned very well with occasional mental health therapy support. However now and then they would lose emotional regulation and become highly reactive in the workplace which resulted in shame and remorse. As their supervisor I named a possible connection to their developmental trauma emotional regulation difficulties within the work context and discussed how they can bolster their support and wellbeing strategies to help get through these times. I did not do therapy with the supervisee (in terms of unpacking these childhood issues with them), but I did help acknowledge the impact of them and help the supervisee recognise signs of unwellness, and access therapy help if they needed this. My focus remained on how these issues were impacting their professional practice and work performance. Hawkins and MacMahon (2020) note that touching on personal aspects of the supervisee should arise from and pertain to work related issues (p. 57). My role was to support critical reflection to increase their insight and self-awareness, and continue to help them build resilience, which supported them to continue to function well in their workplace and provide a high quality service, which they did.

Being able to bring a therapeutic function to supervision reduces the likelihood of workers being 'sent' to therapy to "sort out problematic behaviour" (Krupka, 2014). This is usually from the perspective of the employer who may or may not have adequate insight or awareness of the emotional impacts of the work. Krupka (2014) comments that "If we agree to privilege the working self in supervision, we also need to be aware of not positioning therapy for workers as simply a kind of repair job we recommend in order to get back on the road again". Not being able to hold space for the emotional impacts of human service work in supervision may indicate a supervisor who is fearful of either triggering their own emotional distress or not knowing how to therapeutically respond to the supervisee. This does not mean a worker needs therapy, and messaging this may add to further distress if they feel judged or shamed by the employer or supervisor. If a supervisee is experiencing ongoing distress and this is exacerbated by early life experiences, therapy is a safe and valuable place for a supervisor to suggest. However, therapy should not become an avoidant solution for supervisors, when what may be required is the supervisor's own ability to lean further into the emotional content of what is being shared.

Supervisors who shut down conversations about emotional impacts or fail to open conversations to explore these may also cause supervisees to be selective in what they do and do not share. In research on supervisees' experiences of supervision, O'Donoghue (2012), had a research participant comment that their supervisor's inability to discuss an emotionally upsetting event (and who changed the subject) caused them to then bring superficial issues only to supervision (p. 223). This rendered their supervision inadequate and unsatisfactory. It is likely the supervisor themselves was overwhelmed in some way and not receiving professional supervision where their own emotional responses could be processed and integrated. As supervisors, we will not be able to provide emotional containment for supervisee's experiences if we are not having the space or time to integrate our own. This is not a reason to choose not to engage the therapeutic function of supervision, rather it is a symptom of a lack of reflective space and professional support for ourselves.

Providing an intentional therapeutic function of supervision also invites a softening of rigid boundaries around only work based conversations, it is ok to talk about personal impacts outside of work particularly if these are distressing. The professional role is likely one of many that a person has within a much wider social system. Supervision must allow space for the person who is the professional and recognise they are living multifaceted lives with numerous life experiences. I have had supervisees come into supervision and start crying about a loss of a loved one or a relationship break up. It is not appropriate in these moments to ask for their professional agenda for the session! Instead, I provide a safe supportive therapeutic space that helps them be able to continue where possible with their day. Sometimes the simple act of supporting a distressed supervisee to give themselves permission to go home or take the time they need is the most therapeutic action I can offer.

Ethical considerations

The supervision contract provides an ideal place to name, establish and explore the therapeutic function and the parameters of this. Failing to do this raises ethical issues of not fully informing (leading to confusion) and potentially leaving the supervisee emotionally vulnerable. This includes discussing with the supervisee as to where they would access support outside of supervision if more deep-seated personal issues become triggered. Identifying where personal issues can be worked through also helps make explicit the therapeutic and therapy boundary.

Engaging the therapeutic function of supervision requires a transparent conversation in the getting to know and contracting process that emotional impacts will be explored as part of a therapeutic and reflective process. If time is not taken to inform supervisees of this, they may be unprepared or confused by a supervisor engaging in reflection on the emotional content of the work. This could send the supervision down a therapy/counselling pathway, and even that it be perceived as a friendship, both of which are difficult to return from.

A supervisor should always only work with the scope of their existing skills, and knowledge limitations and not attempt therapeutic interventions which they are not trained in. This requires being explicit about the limits of their experience and knowledge and not engaging in experimental practice that could create harm. Consent to try a new skill in supervision can be a positive learning experience for both supervisee and supervisor but the supervisor must not over-extend or claim skills they do not have. This links to the ethical consideration of committing to ongoing learning in your own supervisory practice, to ensure it is safe, responsible, transparent, and accountable.

In summary, the ethical considerations of applying a therapeutic function in supervision include:

- Preparing the supervisee for the different functions of supervision including the therapeutic function and what this pertains to.
- Establishing what exists outside of supervision to support their wellbeing and should further deeper emotional work be needed.
- Always acting within the bounds of existing skills and not claiming knowledge or practice that may result in harm if poorly delivered.
- Committing to ongoing learning and upskilling to benefit the supervisee and ultimately those they work with.

Ethically applying an intentional therapeutic function in supervision requires attention to all these areas, and in doing this, brings both clarity and commitment to the supervisory relationship, and the roles and responsibilities that set the boundaries within this.

Summary

Line management, clinical and professional supervision all have a valid and important role in the professional and personal development of workers. By clearly defining these and understanding the functions within each, workers can be optimally supported to undertake their roles within the organisation, develop key practice skills and knowledge, and fully integrate their range of experiences into learning and knowledge. The role of the supervisor in professional supervision is to facilitate a critically reflective relational space that includes attending to the emotional content and impacts of the work being undertaken. The supervisee's role is to fully participate actively in the process and being able to critically examine experience for learning.

Engaging the therapeutic function within professional supervision helps support emotional self-awareness and knowledge and contributes to developing resilience to future emotional impacts of human service work. Its overall intention is to support service delivery. It is not a therapist relationship but the application of specific skills to help supervisees process and learn from the emotional impacts of the work. To do this, the supervisor must be able to stand clearly and strongly in the supervisory role and not confuse this with that of their own profession. The supervisor and supervisee relationship is clearly distinct from that of a therapist and client, and this will be further explored in the next chapter. The therapeutic function must be applied in a considered and ethical manner, with transparency as to how and why the supervisor would engage it.

References

Beddoe, L., & Davys, A. (2016). *Challenges in professional supervision: Current themes and models for practice*. London: Jessica Kingsley Publishers.

Beinart, H., & Clohessy, S. (2017). *Effective supervisory relationships: Best evidence and practice*. West Sussex: John Wiley & Sons.

Bond, M., & Holland, S. (2011). *Skills of clinical supervision for nurses: A practical guide for supervisees, clinical supervisors and managers*. Berkshire: McGraw-Hill Education.

28 *Defining the therapeutic function of supervision*

Carroll, M. (2011). Supervision: A journey of lifelong learning. In R. Shohet (Ed.), *Supervision as transformation: A passion for learning* (pp. 14–28). London: Jessica Kingsley Publishers.

Carroll, M. (2014). *Effective supervision for the helping professions.* London: SAGE Publications.

Casement, P. (1985). *On learning from the patient.* London: Tavistock.

Davys, A., & Beddoe, L. (2020). *Best practice in professional supervision: A guide for the helping professions.* 2nd Edition. London. Jessica Kingsley Publishers.

Davys, A., Fouché, C., & Beddoe, L. (2021). Mapping effective interprofessional supervision practice. *The Clinical Supervisor, 40*(2), 179–199.

Ferguson, H. (2018). How social workers reflect in action and when and why they don't: The possibilities and limits to reflective practice in social work. *Social Work Education, 37*(4), 415–442.

Fook, J. (2015). Reflective practice and critical reflection. In J. Lishman (Ed.), *Handbook for practice learning in social work and social care: Knowledge and theory* (pp. 440–454). London: Jessica Kingsley Publishing.

Hawkins, P., & McMahon, A. (2020). *Supervision in the helping professions.* 5th Edition. Open University Press.

Hawkins, P., & Shohet, R. (2012). *Ebook: Supervision in the helping professions.* Berkshire: McGraw-Hill Education.

Herkt, J., & Hocking, C. (2007). Supervision in New Zealand: Professional growth or maintaining competence? *New Zealand Journal of Occupational therapy, 34*(2), 24–30.

Hughes, L., & Pengelly, P. (1997). *Staff supervision in a turbulent environment: Managing process and task in front-line services.* London: Jessica Kingsley Publishers.

Ingham, R. (2021). Emotionally sensitive supervision. In K. O'Donoghue, & L. Engelbrecht (Eds.), *The Routledge international handbook of social work supervision* (pp. 462–471). London: Routledge International.

Itzhaky, H., & Itzhaky, T. (1996). The therapy-supervision dialectic. *Clinical Social Work Journal, 24*, 77–88. DOI: 10.1007/BF02189943.

Kadusshin, A., & Harkness, D. (2014). *Supervision in social work.* New York: Columbia University Press.

Karvinen-Niinikoski, S., Beddoe, L., Ruch, G., & Tsui, M.-S. (2019). Professional supervision and professional autonomy. *Aotearoa New Zealand Social Work, 31*(3), 87+. https://link.gale.com/apps/doc/A673188029/AONE?u=learn&sid=bookmark-AONE&xid=0fd54924.

Knapman, J., & Morrison, T. (1998). *Making the most of supervision in health and social care. A self-development manual for supervisees.* Shoreham-by-Sea: Pavillon.

Krupka, Z. (2014). Therapy in supervision: Responsibility and relationship. *Psychotherapy and Counselling Journal of Australia, 2*(1). https://pacja.org.au/2014/07/therapy-in-supervision-responsibility-and-relationship/

Morrison, T. (1993). *Staff supervision in social care.* London. Longman.

Miller, B. C. (2018). Indirect trauma-sensitive supervision in child welfare. In V. C. Strand, & G. Sprang (Eds.), *Trauma responsive child welfare systems* (pp. 299–314). Springer International Publishing/Springer Nature. DOI: 10.1007/978-3-319-64602-2_19.

O'Donoghue, K. (2012). Windows on the supervisee experience: An exploration of supervisees' supervision histories. *Australian Social Work, 65*(2), 214–231. DOI: 10.1080/0312407X.2012.667816.

O'Donoghue, K. (2021). Advancing the social work supervision research agenda. In K. O'Donoghue, & L. Engelbrecht (Eds.), *The Routledge international handbook of social work supervision* (pp. 637–656). London: Routledge International.

Page, S., & Wosket, V. (2015). *Supervising the counsellor and psychotherapist: A cyclical model.* 3rd Edition. Routledge. DOI: 10.4324/9781315761305.

Paulin, V. (2010). Professional supervision in dietetics: a focus group study investigating New Zealand dietitians' understanding and experience of professional supervision and their perception of its value in dietetic practice. *Nutrition & Dietetics, 67*(2), 106–111. DOI: 10.1111/j.1747-0080.2010. 01428.x

Proctor, B. (1987). Supervision: A co-operative exercise in accountability. In M. Marken, & M. Payne (Eds.), *Enabling and ensuring: Supervision in practice* (pp. 21–34). Leister: National Youth Bureau and the Council for Education and Training in Youth and Community Work.

Rankine, M. (2021). *Thinking critically. A four layered practice model in supervision.* In K. O'Donoghue, & L. Engelbrecht (Eds.), *The Routledge international handbook of social work supervision* (pp. 345–357). London: Routledge International.

Richards, M., & Payne, C. (1990). *Staff supervision in child protection work.* London: National Institute for Social Work.

Ruch, G. (2005). Reflective practice in contemporary child care social work: The role of containment. *British Journal of Social Work, 37*(4), 659–680.

Schamess, G. (2006). Transference enactments in clinical supervision. *Clinical Social Work Journal, 34*(4), 407–425.

Shohet, R. (Ed.) (2011). *Supervision as transformation: A passion for learning.* London: Jessica Kingsley Publishers

Thorpe, K. (2004). Reflective learning journals: From concept to practice. *Reflective Practice, 5*(3), 327–343.

Tripathi, G. (2005). http://socialworkbhu.blogspot.co.nz/2015/04/the-supportive-techniques-in-counselling.html. Downloaded 14 March 2016.

Turney, D., & Ruch, G. (2018). What makes it so hard to look and to listen? Exploring the use of the cognitive and affective supervisory approach with children's social work managers. *Journal of Social Work Practice, 32*(2), 125–138. DOI: 10.1080/02650533.2018.1439460.

Webber-Dreadon, E. (2020). Kaitiakitanga: A transformation of supervision. *Aotearoa New Zealand Social Work, 32*(3), 68–79. DOI: 10.11157/ anzswj-vol32iss3id770.

2 Relational skills to enable the therapeutic function

The enactment of the therapeutic function occurs in a professional supervision relationship where qualities such as trust, warmth, sensitivity, humour, safety, courage, humility, compassion, curiosity, honesty, interest, empathy, openness, mutual respect, and a commitment to reciprocity of learning are present. Interestingly, these qualities mirror some of those identified as required in trauma informed practice, which Levenson (2017) articulates as safety, trust, collaboration, choice, a focus on strengths, and empowerment. Beddoe (2017) comments from her research that supervisors who are warm and engaged but willing to challenge are regarded by supervisees to provide excellent supervision (p. 91). Supervisors also need to have sensitivity to cultural difference and diversity, and awareness of discrimination and inequity.

Beginning with a description on the establishing of a supervisory relationship, this chapter will explore the relational skills of presence, attuning, listening deeply, enabling vulnerability, and applying cultural humility to also support the therapeutic function of supervision.

Developing the supervisory relationship

Positioned within the work and professional context, the heart of professional supervision is the relationship that exists between supervisor and supervisee. The relationship is a partnership, formalised through a contract or supervision agreement to support professional development and quality service delivery. This partnership offers overt learning through what is being outwardly discussed, along with covert learning gained through the experience of the relationship itself and how this can contribute to practice (Loganbill, Hardy & Delworth, 1982). This might include how the supervisor models

DOI: 10.4324/9781003359036-3

responding or thinking about a situation, and the skills they apply to engage with the supervisee. The supervisor also learns from the supervisee, especially across the broad domains of culture and inter-disciplinary supervision, which can support their supervisory and professional practice.

Before beginning a supervisory relationship, time must be taken to get to know the other person. Ideally the supervisee should have a choice of a supervisor, where they have a say about who they'd like to choose. Having a choice can help mitigate some of the inherent power imbalance present in supervision. O'Donoghue (2012) noted that supervisees who had a choice of supervisor and also the supervisor being external to the agency, 'used supervision more purposefully to meet their needs and they displayed a greater personal professional openness and trust in the process and relationship' (p. 222).

To begin the process of getting to know each other, the inviting and sharing of each one's professional journey begins to build understanding and connection. This is followed by asking about the supervisee's experience of supervision, and what has been helpful and also what has not. If a person is new to supervision, this provides a space for the supervisor to explain what professional supervision is. It is here that the supervisee can share their hopes for supervision which may include sharing learning needs and how they best learn.

The supervisor then shares their supervisory journey, how it looks currently, and particular approaches or theories they apply in their supervisory practice. This is also a good place for the supervisor to identify any potential conflicts of interest, such as supervising others in the service or agency, and whether this will be workable for the supervisee.

The supervisee can then reflect if what the supervisor is offering will best meet their learning needs and hopes, while the supervisor can consider if they have the skills for what the supervisee is looking for. Throughout this process both parties assess whether a productive and supportive supervisory relationship can be established, essentially the provision of a 'safe base' to enable exploration (Carroll, 2014; Beinart & Clohessy, 2017, p. 32). The overall intention in the getting to know phase can be summarised as determining whether enough relational comfort to enable the sometimes uncomfortable act of criti-cal reflection can be established, essentially being comfortable enough to get uncomfortable.

In this early development of a potential supervisory relationship, both parties are guided by how each other communicates. Noticeable barriers in communication, high points of difference or points of disconnect in this first meeting may indicate that the relationship will not develop well. Openness about any other limitations or barriers including cultural difference and commonality is very helpful here, with a balance of both likely to indicate the potential for security and learning. An example of this might be someone who works in a church-based organisation where they are also a member of that church, while the supervisor is an atheist so does not share their beliefs. While it may not be an issue, it is best surfaced at this stage and discussed. Honesty and transparency as this stage sets the scene for a productive working relationship that can be then formally contracted if the decision is to proceed.

The contract will contain agreement about frequency of meeting, confidentiality (and the limits to this), management of conflict, and related organisational or professional mandates pertaining to supervision. These might include responsibilities such as payment, recording, and reviews of the supervision relationship, and required reports. Time is then taken to identify how the supervisor and supervisee will commit to working together, including expectations for the working relationship. This will likely include discussing responsibilities around agenda setting, how to best attend to learning styles, and communication commitments, for example, how to constructively both give and receive feedback.

Within the getting to know each and contracting phase, the place of the therapeutic function of supervision can be articulated, which is easily done by explaining the three core functions of supervision and expanding on the restorative. This would also include differentiating between therapeutic and therapy so there is no confusion about this. Transparency around the attention to the emotional impacts of the work and support of worker wellbeing and safety of practice will allow the supervisee and supervisor to confidently move into the therapeutic function as required. With this understanding in place, the following skills can then be applied at any time in supervision but especially to apply the therapeutic function.

Presence

Described by Senge, Scharmer, Jaworski, and Flowers (2005) through Scharmer's 'U' theory, the notion of 'presence' contains the concepts of sensing, presencing, and realising. The first side of the 'U' is about letting go, putting aside previous notions and thinking, and from here moving downward into deepening and opening into learning. The bottom of the 'U' is where someone is fully present and aware.

Once present we can then begin to move up the other side of the 'U', to let come, so opening ourselves up to insights and discoveries with the intention of moving these into action. Similar to the Kolb (1984) experiential learning, cycle (discussed in the next chapter), it invites movement into being (reflection) and then up and outward into action. It invites us to move from the activity of doing into the stillness of being, and then gently outward back to doing.

Presence is also articulated through the Māori concept of 'Wātea', a state of being free of what has happened before and entering the present moment (Moorfield, 2011). It involves a silencing and stilling of one's own emotions and thoughts. It opens a space that is offered with the intention of "I am here to bear witness to your journey and your story, I am unencumbered, I am free to be in this space with you, I am committed to focus and attend to you today and journey with you in exploring and learning".

For me this is a very intentional process that begins before I arrive in the supervision space. I bring to mind the person I am about to have supervision with and connect with their energy and life force that I have awareness of. I focus on what I enjoy about them, what I already know, and the invitation to learn more about who they are and the work they do. I connect to the privilege of being on their professional journey with them, and also acknowledge and bring to mind how this can at times feel vulnerable for them.

I also mentally put down whatever I might be carrying from the day or week by reminding myself of this being their time, a small space usually once a month, that is for their personal and professional development. When I see them, I smile, make eye contact, I may make a small talk, just to help them adjust to being in my presence again and also to convey that it is a non-threatening and safe space we are co-creating. It is very important I make obvious my pleasure at seeing them again. Rodgers (2011) comments that, "In therapy and supervision we come together in the hope of being truly seen" (p. 105). The simple act of conveying seeing, is a critical vein that runs through the heart of the therapeutic function, and it begins on the very first point of re-engagement. I am already noticing the supervisee's energy, reading body and voice cues for how they might be feeling today, and what they might need to settle into being, reflecting, exploring, and learning.

Once we are seated and small re-engaging chat is exchanged, I smile, pause, and begin with an enquiry as to how they are doing, how their week or day is going. If there is high emotionality occurring, I gently check if it would be helpful to talk that through, or if they seem ok, I ask what they would like to explore or reflect on today and what would be helpful from our time together in regard to this. Once we begin talking, I remain conscious of this stage being about a place of naming and letting go, a space for them to tell me what is happening or happened, all the while being aware of inviting them to go deeper into the reflection and thinking.

When it is apparent the issue is one of higher emotional content, I consciously move into the therapeutic function. This begins with my own stilling of emotional energy, quieting of my thoughts, and leaning into what is being shared through giving it my full attention. As someone with a busy curious mind, I use breath to ensure I am grounded, I lengthen my exhaled breath to help settle myself, and I sometimes put my feet more firmly on the floor to deliberately anchor and not let distraction enter. It is a highly conscious and intentional use of my body and my mind to be fully present with them. Sometimes I even say in my mind "be still, be present, be quiet, be here" so my attention is fully with them.

If I am fully present, then I can intentionally help the supervisee to also be, and therefore engage in and complete the task of letting go and letting come. I am aligning, while not necessarily joining, with their emotional state. I am offering a calm regulated presence that offers reassurance and acceptance of what they wish to share.

Attuning

Presence enables the inherent process of attuning and attending to the supervisee that flows throughout the session. Schamess (2006) comments that supervision is "most effective when it creates a holding environment that enhances empathetic attunement and relational capacity" (p. 433). The quality of attuning is the foundation to professional supervision as everything builds and develops from this skill. Within the reconnecting phase of supervision, there is a determining of the emotional state of the supervisee, which is elicited by reading body language, enquiring, and noticing changes to the person's usual demeanor or state. This requires a specific form of listening that pays attention to a wide range of cues and brings the supervisor's full attention to the supervisee. The beginning phase of attuning signals that this time is a protected space for the supervisee to be themselves and explore what is foremost for them. Whatever may have been happening for the supervisor in their own day is now put to one side and the conscious application of attention begins.

Over two consecutive days I entered the supervision space with different supervisees and was immediately aware of a lower energy level emanating from them than what was usual. The first person presented as quieter and sad, the second, in response to my opening question of "How are you doing?" smiled tentatively and said "Ok" in a hesitant manner, which immediately gave me a clue that something was emotionally pressing for them. With the first person when I asked that question, they shared they didn't want to be at work, and everything was feeling 'really hard'. As part of my attuning and noticing I moved into holding space for what might come. I postponed developing a structured agenda, so replaced my usual question of "What would be helpful from our time together today?" with enquiring if they would like to explore that feeling of 'everything was really hard'.

By attuning to a person's emotional state, I signal acceptance and safety for whatever they may want to bring forward. I notice a stilling and sometimes a 'turning down' of my own emotional energy level, namely if I have arrived in a high energy space. Essentially, I begin a degree of matching but not joining with the supervisee's emotional state. I attune and use an acknowledging question of "I can see something may be happening or has happened that is feeling hard. Is that right?" This provides an open invitation for them to move into sharing whatever they feel comfortable with.

With the first person, I had a relatively new supervisory relationship, and while they acknowledged something personal had happened, they were protective of this and instead wanted to engage in a more work-based conversation which we tried for a little while. I could sense a sadness and a difficulty in engaging with what we were discussing so I put my pen down on my recording sheet. I named that they had said at the beginning they didn't really want to be at work that day, and I was wondering if they had much energy for talking about work. Attuning requires a delicate dance of respecting a boundary or line over which a person may not be ready to step, but also honouring and responding to the emotionality that is present. People may not want to step across this line for fear of moving into an emotionally unrecoverable space, or just from being very private or feeling too fragile or vulnerable. Therapeutic support can still occur without knowing the specific detail of the upsetting event, although a general context can be helpful.

In the first session, my focus became how I can assist in providing a restorative space, convey positive regard to gently strengthen, and develop a degree of structured planning to assist them to be feeling ready to meet their professional duties that day. This highlights another difference between supervision and therapy. As a therapist I may have been explored deeper into what was happening personally, as a supervisor I had a duty of care to their clients.

With the second person, I had a long-established relationship with high trust, and this person was able to move freely into discussing the impacts of an unfolding new life event that was pulling their focus away from work. I continued to hold the same intention of restoring and strengthening, knowing this conversation, while located strongly in a personal context, would free them to be more available in their work. I provided space for their narrative to be shared and asked questions that helped them come to place where some anxiety and tension could be released. In this session I was able to be a little more directive in my responses, as we were building off previously explored areas of their emotional management.

Listening deeply

A supervisory relationship that is attuned and supports presence requires what I call 'whole of self' listening. To undertake the therapeutic function of supervision, the skills of listening are turned up higher. There are words to be heard, but it is the tone of the words and the body movements that accompany them that are also being observed and listened to. It is not just with my ears that I am listening, it is a whole of person noticing that I am engaging in.

I am listening for the feelings that need a voice, the thoughts that want to be heard but worry about being judged, and the fears that hold these within. I am listening to the shifts in body language, the looking away, the nervous laugh, the tears that may be sitting close to the surface of the eyes, and to the anger that wants expression. I lean in and give permission through conveying non-judgement that all of these emotions can be expressed and accepted in our space together.

Listening ultimately supports being heard, which is the first step in the process of restoring and strengthening. To be truly listened to enables us to feel seen. I convey my listening through gentle eye contact, giving space to this as needed, through nodding, simple affirming and acknowledging words, summarising, paraphrasing, and conveying my full attention. I use curiosity and wondering to keep my attention and listening tuned in and amplified especially for supervisees who have come from childhood histories of abuse and neglect, where their sensitivity to non-verbal cues is heightened.

I also remain aware that given the limited time frame of supervision, we will need to surface out at some stage and that they need to be ok to head back into their day. I listen for the lighting of emotion and ask questions to support the re-emergence into the workspace. Deeper listening can sometimes be the only thing we can offer in times where there are no easy solutions but being truly listened to and heard can restore enough energy to keep going.

Enabling vulnerability

Undertaking the therapeutic function of supervision does require a supervisee at times to be able to open into vulnerability. This can only occur in a relationship of trust and without fear of repercussion or blaming or judgement. A key to enabling vulnerability is the conveying of unconditional positive regard and acceptance. We will not enter vulnerability with people we do not feel this from. Workers may worry, as do supervisors, that they will lose control emotionally and may avoid talking about emotions for fear of this. There may also be a worry of being perceived as 'not coping' which I counter with the high expression of emotion often being a sign of trying to cope. As supervisors, we must also convey that we are capable and able to contain and hold strong emotions or vulnerability, and this is again signalled by the quality of attuned presence we create and also being calm and regulated in ourselves.

A key to enabling vulnerability is the way we recognise, acknowledge, and respond to the expression of it in the supervision session. Simple acknowledgement such as "That sounds really hard", "I'm so sorry you had that experience", or "Thank you for sharing that with me" not only show that we have listened but that we have heard and are emotionally responding back. We can share a simple sentence of how what they have shared has touched us such as, "I could feel myself experiencing something of the sadness you have shared" or "I found myself imagining how that might have been, and noticed a tightening in myself, is that how it was for you?" This notion of 'resonating' indicates that we have leaned into the experience but are still steady and present (Fairfield, 2013). It is a validating, affirming, and normalising of the experience. This reduces the feeling of sometimes being alone or feeling isolated through what is happening or has happened.

Emotional based questions help surface vulnerability in the supervisory relationship. The simple question of "How are you feeling right now talking about this?" can help move a person deeper into the process of letting go and being present. Another question is "Where are you noticing that feeling in your body?" to help a person move into noticing where the feeling might be creating tension or strain in their body. The 'one word answer' is another useful way to help people move into reflection, and by locating this to feeling helps give their emotions voice. So, "If you could name with just one word how you are feeling [or how you felt] what would that be?" we can then ask for greater detail about that word and help them explore the thoughts that might come with it and the connected reactions or behaviours it might bring. For some people this enquiry is more personal and can feel more vulnerable, but it will also support self-awareness and expression, therefore contributing to greater integration and learning. There are a range of other ways to work with the emotional content in supervision which will be explored in Chapter 5.

The types of questions applied invite the supervisee into deeper emotional reflection and as a supervisor we gauge the extent with which to take this, again respecting we are not therapists, in the context of a supervisory relationship. It is noticing the opportunity to invite a supervisee into a deeper reflection and enquiry, to which I provide quiet and stillness, and sometimes a question that they can continue to reflect on.

An example of this was a supervisee sharing they felt uncomfortable at times in their work when it was quiet, and they were not so busy. They named feeling an unease in these times and a worry they were not doing enough. I asked what emotion or thoughts they had at these times which they struggled to answer. I asked if it was a worry, an uncomfortableness, perhaps they felt restless? They shared that that it was a worry that they would be seen as not being a hard worker and that they should be doing something. We discussed a reframe that these times could be seen as restoring and helped accumulate more energy for times when the work increased again. The supervisee could easily grasp this intellectually, but I sensed a barrier to allowing herself to fully accept or permit it. I named I was observing a slight hesitance around giving themselves permission for this.

I suggested that perhaps in these times they could gently speak back to the thoughts that began with "I should". I wondered if it might help to notice if there is another voice underlying those thoughts such as an inner critic which could be from other times in their life. They looked thoughtful and I then said we can speak back to the message to be highly driven and 'doing' at all times by consciously thinking, "I am enough". They gave a small physical jolt when I said this, and that was far enough to take the conversation at that time. Sometimes leaving a person with something to consider and reflect on, a seed that is sown, enables a continuation of therapeutic strengthening and a potential transformative moment.

Enabling vulnerability supports the concepts of the Johari window developed by Jospeh Luft and Harrington Ingham in 1955. The Johari window observes that there are four panes through which we can recognise and increase knowledge happening between two people. One pane is that what is known and understood by both, including freely available and shared role and demographical information. There is a pane that is blind, so known to the observer but not the other person. An example of this would be unaware physical tensing, unconscious patterns of emotional response, or fidgeting or holding of an unconscious bias. Another pane relates to knowledge that is hidden, so information a person knows about themselves, but they may not be ready or willing to share. This could include mental health challenges or sexual identity. Finally, the unknown pane is knowledge both are yet to experience. Supervision should provide a safe space for hidden details to be revealed once trust is developed, and for blind information to be respectfully surfaced as appropriate. The unknown space becomes an invitation to participate in a continuous point of growth and learning for both.

If a supervisee has entered vulnerability with us, we have a responsibility to ensure they are in an ok place by the end of the session so they can return to work. As our time comes to an end, we can ask a question such as "Can I just check how you are feeling right now?" which helps us to know where they are now at. We can encourage them to make a plan if they feel unable to return to work and discover how we can support them in this. Thanking and acknowledging people for what has been shared, and articulating any learning for ourselves can help shift a person back into work mode. Gentle humour, noticing emerging events outside of the room such as lunch time or the comings and goings of others can help bring them into being ready to re-engage. Making another supervision time, offering that this can be sooner than originally scheduled if they wish, and checking back around what they will do now the session is over also help ground and reorientate people. We are now on the other side of the 'U' and heading back into the world. To be vulnerable with someone relies on knowing they are present, attentive to us, and that they care.

Cultural humility

Culture is a broad term encompassing ethnicity, religion, socio-economic status, politics, sexuality, disability, gender, and spiritual beliefs. It can be evidenced through customs, behaviours, values, ancestral stories, and language (Tsui, O'Donoghue & Ng, 2014) and informs our identity. In addition every person has their own culture shaped by the families they grew up in and the wider environments of society, and country. Our choice of profession and the culture inherent in that will also influence how we respond to different situations.

For populations who have experienced the devastation of colonisation, slavery, genocide, and ostracisation from society, the restoration of culture followed by preservation of this is essential. While the past cannot be undone, learning from it helps build a different future. Supervision must contribute to repair and restoration where once silenced voices get to speak again, and where what is shared is carefully held and respected. It is not words alone that build repair, it is actions.

For supervision to be a safe relational space for cultural difference, supervisors must engage in an ongoing journey of learning to work cross culturally, so recognising and responding to the interrelated personal, cultural, and professional domains of the supervisee (Su'a-Hawkins & Mafile'o, 2004, p. 15). This includes holding a clear intention to open conversations that invite interpersonal exchanges that explore and integrate similarities and differences.

Cultural humility is a concept that underlies the notion of cultural responsiveness, by articulating an interpersonal way of being with people (Hook et al., 2016). This includes an awareness of one's own cultural limitations and bias developed from socialisation experiences and the demonstration of a lifelong commitment to learning, self-examination and self-critique. Hook et al, identify cultural humility as evidencing a humbleness about one's own limitations and recognising a lack of knowledge or understanding. This also includes developing awareness of majority culture privilege and taking steps in addressing the inequity inherent in this. Cultural humility gives space for different voices to be heard through an intention of inclusion, moving to a position of not knowing, and a commitment to listening and learning.

A supervisor with cultural humility is self-aware, with an attitude of openness and transparency, and has respectful curiosity around cultural difference where they actively seek to understand different perspectives and learn. Hook et al. (2016) suggest cultural humility initiates conversations about cultural diversity, invites open discussion where their own bias is acknowledged, and through doing this, also helps the supervisee to instill cultural humility in their work with others. They also note there is an ongoing process of assessing one's strengths and weaknesses from our own cultural experiences, building a plan to work proactively on cultural humility, and connecting with diverse population groups to help challenge bias and lack of understanding and build different perspectives (Hook et al., 2016, p. 155).

To engage in this type of interpersonal exchange both demonstrates and celebrates the concept of 'va' from some Pasifika cultures, so honouring the sacred relational space between people, environment, and ancestors. Cultural humility also embraces the concept of 'ako', drawn from Māori wisdom, which upholds reciprocity of learning from each other, where knowledge is socially constructed between both supervisor and supervisee (Hair & O'Donoghue, 2009).

An example of supervising from a place of cultural humility is the experience of working with Māori and the range of Pasifika cultures in Aotearoa, New Zealand around the notion of 'self-care'. Cultural norms across these ethnicities tend to prioritise immediate and extended family before the individual, so rather than a concept of 'I' there is a foundation of 'we'. Without seeking to understand a collectivist lens, a conversation of supporting individual wellbeing is not likely to land very well and could create a sense of dissonance within the supervisee. Instead, an exploration around how supporting wellbeing in others along with ourselves may be a more effective approach. Building understanding by questions such as "I'm feeling aware that suggestion comes from my cultural lens, could you help me understand how that might be from your perspective?" help reduce difficulty in communication and misunderstandings.

Power and authority may also be factors that need to be understood and surfaced from a perspective of cultural humility. Tsui, O'Donoghue and Ng (2014) note that collectivist cultures tend to respect and follow group norms with a greater emphasis on position and authority. If a supervisee comes from a collectivist culture where challenging or speaking up seemingly against a person in perceived authority is discouraged, then the imbalance of power inherent within a supervisory relationship may be more greatly accentuated. Therefore, disagreeing or debating with the supervisor is less likely to occur which may create internal conflict for a supervisee who may not agree or feels unable to act on a particular course of action.

The supervisor needs to ensure space occurs for the supervisee to be able to voice difficulties in a way that remains respectful for them and invite exploration of their willingness, capacity, and confidence in what is being suggested. The supervisor can transparently name "I realise it might feel hard to disagree with me, but I'm very open to this" or "As I'm not from your culture, please feel able tell me if that would work or not, this would very much help my learning". Cultural humility involves 'not knowing' and committing to exploring intersectionality to increase knowledge and understanding. The relational qualities of trust, respect, interest, curiosity, appreciation, and warmth essential to professional supervision all contribute to cultural humility.

It is also essential that as supervisors we utilise our own supervision to explore and unpack unconscious bias from our own life journey. We also need to ensure that the supervision space we provide is a safe space where the supervisee knows this can be critically examined. I had an example of this in relation to unconscious gender bias where a supervisee reflected that they had minimised bullying behaviour from a group of boys toward a girl, saying to her that it was probably as a sign they might like her. My supervisee was horrified when they reflected on this, seeing it as potentially contributing to possible normalising of violence in future intimate relationships for the girl. They recognised that they had been given this type of justification as a young person and had unconsciously formed a gender bias. We discussed how socialisation contributes to such comments and the importance of being able to realise and make these conscious. We also rehearsed how they would respond in the future and the possibility of working with children to also explore these sort of social messages.

It is impossible to emerge from our own journeys of socialisation without collecting cultural bias, and if from a majority culture, privilege. It requires an intentional lifelong commitment to notice, explore, and replace this with cultural humility. This helps self-learning and the development of social narratives that uphold the rights and dignity for all. Cultural humility requires respectful and thoughtful attention to acceptance and understanding with an underlying commitment to equity and recognition of bias and discrimination both societally and internally. As supervisors we commit to a life long journey of cultural humility and continue to explore our own lack of knowledge and areas of unconscious and conscious judgment in our own supervision.

Summary

The supervisor relationship is the vehicle within which the therapeutic function can occur. A supervisory relationship that supports the therapeutic function is one that ultimately conveys the message of "I see you". It begins with attuning, observing and noticing immediately on re-engagement. The application of presence and wātea provide the conditions for this and assists the supervisee to be present and able to move through a reflective journey of being with what is and allowing space for what could be. This safe space for the therapeutic function in supervision requires 'whole of self' listening that leans into the emotional world of the supervisee as required. This enables and supports vulnerability to surface which supports deeper reflection, insight, and self-discovery. The relational space we develop must demonstrate a commitment to cultural humility, where the supervisor is engaged in lifelong learning of both unpacking their own culture, able to 'not know' and demonstrating a willingness to learn.

References

Beddoe, L. (2017). Harmful supervision: A commentary. *The Clinical Supervisor, 36*(1), 88–101. DOI: 10.1080/07325223.2017.1295894.

Beinart, H., & Clohessy, S. (2017). *Effective supervisory relationships: Best evidence and practice.* West Sussex: John Wiley & Sons.

Carroll, M. (2014). *Effective supervision for the helping professions.* London: SAGE Publications.

Fairfield, M. (2013). The Relational movement. British Gestalt Journal. Vol. 22. No. 1. pp 22–35.

Hair, H., & O'Donoghue, K. (2009) Culturally relevant, socially just social work supervision: Becoming visible through a social constructionist lens. *Journal of Ethnic & Cultural Diversity in Social Work, 18*(1–2), 70–88. DOI: 10.1080/15313200902874979.

Hook, J. N., Watkins, C. E., Davis, D. E., Owen, J., Van Tongeren, D. R., & Ramos, M. J. (2016). Cultural humility in psychotherapy supervision. *American Journal of Psychotherapy, 70*(2), 149–166. DOI: 10.1176/appi.psychotherapy.2016.70.2.149.

Kolb, D. (1984). *Experiential learning as the source of learning and development.* Englewood Cliffs, NJ: Prentice Hall.

Loganbill, C., Hardy, E., & Delworth, U. (1982). Supervision: A conceptual model. *The Counseling Psychologist, 10*(1), 3–42. DOI: 10.1177/0011000082101002.

Levenson, J. (2017). Trauma-informed social work practice. *Social Work, 62*(2), 105–113.

Luft, J., & Ingham, H. (1955). The Johari window; A graphic model of interpersonal awareness. In *Proceedings of the Western training laboratory in group development.* Los Angeles, CA, UCLA Extension Office.

Moorfield, J. (2011). *Te Aka Māori-English, English-Māori dictionary and index.* Auckland: Longman/Pearson Education.

O'Donoghue, K. (2012). Windows on the supervisee experience: An exploration of supervisees' supervision histories. *Australian Social Work, 65*(2), 214–231. DOI: 10.1080/0312407X.2012.667816.

Rodgers, A. (2011). Supervision through conversation: Being seen, being real. In R. Shohet (Ed.), *Supervision as transformation: A passion for learning* (pp. 106–122). London: Jessica Kingsley Publishers.

Schamess, G. (2006). Transference enactments in clinical supervision. *Clinical Social Work Journal, 34*(4), 407–425.

Senge, P., Scharmer, O. C., Jaworski, J., & Flowers, B. S. (2005). *Presence: Exploring profound change in people, organisations and society.* London: Nicholas Brealey Publishing.

Su'a-Hawkins, A., & Mafile'o, T. (2004). What is cultural supervision? *Social Work Now, 29*, 10–16.

Tsui, M.-s., O'Donoghue, K., & Ng, A. K. T. (2014). Culturally competent and diversity-sensitive clinical supervision: An international perspective. In C. E. Watkins, Jr., & D. L. Milne (Eds.), *The Wiley international handbook of clinical supervision* (pp. 238–254). Wiley-Blackwell. DOI: 10.1002/9781118846360.ch10.

3 Developing a coherent narrative

When working with experiences of distress, trauma, and indirect trauma impacts, supporting the supervisee to tell the story of what has happened or is happening is the first step to integrate the experience. Integration of the experience helps prevent further emotional difficulty from it which may continue to cause distress. Experiences that are not integrated, especially those with high emotional content, can continue to have impacts such as rumination, self-doubt, loss of confidence and cognitive intrusion. Left unattended, these can contribute to Acute Stress Disorder or Post Traumatic Stress Disorder or Secondary Traumatic Stress.

Bond and Holland (2011) note that instead of counselling or therapy, in times of high distress, the concepts of psychological first aid can be applied. These include: providing relational engagement, enhancing safety and comfort through practical assistance, calming and orienting, providing information, connecting to others or services, promoting/restoring self-efficacy, and restoring hope by identifying action steps that are realistic and help provide structure and a plan. These actions are certainly applicable to the supervision setting in times when coping has been temporarily disrupted, and attending to a supervisee in this way provides a pathway for the development of a coherent narrative.

Trauma Focused Cognitive Behaviour Therapy applies the concept of developing a trauma narrative to helping people to process and integrate what has occurred. This begins by firstly ensuring a person has emotional language and ways of anchoring and self-soothing before the telling of the traumatic event. The development of the trauma narrative helps integrate the experience and move further into memory, reducing the need to return to it. The emotionality of the event is diminished and the risk of it becoming an intrusive memory

DOI: 10.4324/9781003359036-4

is contained. The idea of a developing coherent narrative is a little broader and can be applied to a variety of situations which may be on a continuum of distressing to traumatic. Development of the narrative provides information and knowledge for future situations and enables a supervisee to move on from an experience.

Reflective learning processes

The process of developing a coherent narrative in supervision is underpinned by a reflective process that moves from the telling of what has occurred to learning, developing insight, making meaning, and gaining knowledge that can be applied. Carroll (2009) comments that "reflection is the ability to think about the past, in the present, for the future" (p. 41). Supervision provides an ideal place to develop and engage in reflective practice, holding a wider intention of installing this as a daily skill for practitioners that they can apply to a variety of situations. This was summarised by Schon (1983) as reflection on action and reflection in action.

Hawkins and Shohet (2012) observe four aspects of reflection in supervision – external reflection where the supervisee reflects on what is happening with the client, introspective reflection, where the supervisee reflects on themselves and their thoughts and feelings in relation to the client, this is followed by relational reflection, where the supervisee reflects on the interaction and relationship between themselves and the client, and finally systemic reflection, where the supervisee reflects on the 'wider context or system in which the working relationship is embedded' (p. 17).

The Kolb experiential learning cycle (1984) provides a simple four-stage cyclical model to understand adult learning which can be applied to supervision to support reflective practice (Morrison, 1993). In the concrete experience stage of the model, the supervisee is invited to tell what happened (or what is happening), so describe the issue, and the context in which it occurred. Reflection on the issue then begins, where the supervisee shares their reactions and responses by identifying and exploring their thoughts and feelings. The next stage of abstract conceptualisation is where the supervisee engages in critical reflection to make sense of the issue and their responses to this. This process of meta cognition engages the supervisee in wondering, considering, and analysing their thinking about what occurred. The supervisor might offer their thoughts and hypothesises regarding the situation in a bid to help the supervisee consider other viewpoints to deepen understanding.

Finally, the stage of active experimentation offers the supervisee the chance to integrate the experience into learning by considering what they did well, and what they might do differently. It provides an opportunity to check how the supervisee feels about the situation now, and what their learning is from it. The unpacking and developing of learning gained from the experience can now be applied in the future.

The Reflective Learning Model provided by Davys (2001) emphasises the role of the supervisor not as an expert but as providing the 'space and context for learning' (Davys & Beddoe, 2020, p. 102). It builds on the Kolb learning cycle stages, with in-depth time spent at the beginning to set a clear supervision goal that uncovers the supervisee's dilemma about the issue so not just describing the issue (Davys & Beddoe, 2021). It challenges supervisees to move from a place of all knowing to unknowing and discovery.

By also applying a four-stage process, the first stage (after the initial reconnecting) is the 'Event' where developing clarity of the agenda item that supervisee wishes to reflect and explore, and their hopes/goal for what will be achieved occurs. The process then moves to 'Exploration' a two-stage process of developing perspective on (1) impacts (personal emotional reflection on responses), and (2) implications (analytical cognitive reflection enabling conceptualisation of the issue within the wider organisational and professional context). The issue is reflected on through listening, clarifying, and asking questions to increase awareness and understanding, which locates the supervisee clearly in the issue by examining their thoughts, feelings and assumptions (Davys & Beddoe, 2020).

A plan of action can begin to emerge here which in the 'Experimentation' stage, is tested for clarity, including roles and responsibilities and what else might be needed for the action to be applied to practice. This is where learning is highlighted and what might now be done differently happens. Finally, the 'Evaluation' stage returns to the agenda item to evaluate if the goal stated at the beginning of the session has been reached/resolved, confirming the learning that has occurred, and any other issues that have arisen from it that may require time in the next session. The session is then concluded. Davys and Beddoe (2020) summarise the process as Goal, Reflect, Analyse, Plan and Evaluate – GRAPE.

In another reflective process model, Watkins, Callahan, and Vîşcu (2019) developed the Supervision Session Pyramid, also containing four stages. The base of the pyramid covers the first stage of event issue identification and clarification, the next stage up is exploration and elaboration, this then moves to experimentation and consolidation, and finally review and resolution of the issue. They acknowledge that issues may not be fully resolved in one session but can be resolved to the point of good enough for now. The overall intention to tell, explore, and integrate, is similar to the Kolb stages, beginning with telling the story of what the issue is, moving into deeper reflection on this through the use of skilled questioning, exploring ways to resolve or assist with it, and then determining where the issue is sitting by the end of the supervision session.

All of these reflective process models help supervisees develop clarity, insight, and provide an opportunity to integrate the experience into their practice wisdom and professional development. For the supervisor, applying a reflective learning process helps ensure insight into the worker's practice occurs and not simply a description of what has happened, but also the 'how' and 'why' of this (Thorpe, 2004). It assists with finding our way through the client story to the practice of the worker.

I had a supervisee who had experienced a situation with another professional who had considerable societally sanctioned power and authority and used this to mock and humiliate the supervisee's client. My supervisee had been taken off guard by this unexpected behaviour and was left feeling distressed and angered by it. In our agenda setting, they identified wanting to reduce the emotional impact of the experience and have some strategies to help manage it in the future if it occurred again.

I invited them to tell me what happened and asked probing questions, so the experience was described with as much detail as possible, a technique that helps with the coherence of the narrative. Once they had done this, we then spent time in the reflecting and elaborating on their emotional reaction to what had occurred, which was a combination of shock and anger. I asked them to describe the feelings and where they had noticed them within themselves. I then asked them how they managed these feelings, and they described taking deliberate pauses before speaking, and focusing on a key point to provide advocacy for the client.

In the conceptualisation/exploration stage of the cycle, I asked them what they thought might have been occurring for the other person and we then discussed ways to best manage this type of behaviour including anything they might have done differently in the process leading up to this incident. I asked them if in the future another person with this power status behaved in such a way, how would they feel. They named feeling a little anxious about this, so I asked them to describe how they would like to respond. This now moved us into the active experimentation/consolidation of the learning cycle where learning is identified and steps to move forward outlined.

My supervisee named a partial possible desired future response but stalled a little, so I invited them to think about other colleagues who managed these behaviours well, and what they did. As they talked about this, their energy noticeably lifted, and they started seeing the situation as one of opportunity and challenge in terms of aspiring to respond to it differently. We discussed some initial steps toward this, including continuing to notice, observe and manage their anger both during an incident and after. I concluded by naming what I thought they had done well and then checking with how it was sitting with them now. We then checked whether the session had met their goal at the beginning which they felt it had. The reflective learning process was completed, enabling them to integrate the experience further, have a more coherent narrative for it and their responses to it, and learning from it.

Explore inaccurate thoughts

In helping a supervisee develop a coherent narrative around a situation or event, we need to notice and explore any thoughts or beliefs that are distorted or possibly not accurate. Inaccurate thoughts can prolong the processing of a stressful or distressing situation, by contributing to rumination and emotions such as shame or self-blame. The surfacing of inaccurate thoughts happens in the reflection and the conceptualisation stage of the experiential learning cycle. A clue to this is in the emotional response being described and whether this accurately matches the experience. If the emotional response seems too high in its intensity, it is likely that other experiences, self-beliefs or dilemmas may be layered onto this one. Another indicator is where the supervisee is expressing significant rumination so going over and over the situation, or where they have gone too far forward in their thinking including predicting consequences or outcomes that may not occur.

A way to surface inaccurate thoughts is to gently enquire what the evidence is for them. This returns the conversation to one of facts and reins in layering of additional emotion or speculation. An example would be ruminating on a presentation that had perhaps not gone as well as hoped but now the supervisee is expressing self-blame that they let people down and wasted their time. This type of thinking left unchallenged could contribute into a series of thought looping such as,

That didn't go as well as I hoped, two people seemed bored, oh gosh, everyone must have been bored, I must have been boring, I'm no good at these sorts of presentations, I wasted their time, they'll never ask me back, how could I have got it so wrong, what a nightmare, I can never do a presentation ever again, deep down I'm just a fraud and everyone knows that now. The result of this thought catastrophising is therefore persistent feelings of shame, upset, and self-blame. Exploring the evidence for this would include acknowledging that it sounds like the presentation did not go as well as hoped but the evidence that everyone was bored, and they are now hopeless at presenting is a form of totalising which denies the parts that might have been fine and the people there who were engaged.

Reframing provides a way of offering alternative thinking including providing a different perspective such as "It sounds like you really tried, and doing a good job of the presentation mattered to you, is it possible the brief you were given wasn't clear?" Or, "What do you think are people's responsibilities in learning situations like these?" Hearing another person's views on what has happened brings a different way of looking at the situation and brings objectivity to it. This alternative viewpoint helps challenge inaccurate thoughts and can soften harsh or critical self-judgement. A supervisor is essentially saying "I can hear your view, but I also can hear something different in here". Offering a different perspective invites a different set of emotional responses or reduces the intensity of these.

This is also a way of attributing correct levels of personal responsibility. While there might have been something that could have been done differently in a situation, there can be an over assuming of responsibility and an incorrect attribution of power and influence. This is especially important in traumatising or distressing events where a person may think everything that happened is their fault and they could have stopped or prevented the event. We can acknowledge that it would have been their hope but is not always possible. Ensuring the correct responsibility is assumed can help a supervisee recognise that they are not and cannot be responsible for everything that may have happened, which, in turn, reduces self-blame, rumination, and shame.

Connect to strengths and existing resiliency

Once a supervisee has been given space to tell and reflect on the story, the supervisor can explore previous ways they have managed and how they did this. This solution focused technique of connecting to existing strategies, wisdom, coping, and strengths, serves to surface, apply and reinforce them. Being invited to articulate what they already know and how they apply this, reinforces a person's existing resources. Asking questions and assisting the supervisee to examine it further helps to reinforce and conceptualise what they do know and how they apply it.

I had an example of this with a supervisee who was feeling frustrated, disappointed, and overwhelmed with the existing lack of mental health services. They were finding themselves with highly distressed people for whom they could not access timely mental health support. This is an example of an external persistent societal stressor that is not easily changeable. Societal stressors can cause a worker to join in the feelings of hopelessness, helplessness and overwhelm experienced by their clients. It can also contribute to those feelings arising in a supervisor if we too try and problem solve a complex and somewhat intractable problem. It may also be tempting to join in a criticism of other services contributing to fractured professional networks. While continuing to acknowledge it was indeed frustrating and overwhelming, I invited the supervisee to tell me what they do in those times with people, focusing firstly on people who are very heightened and anxious and then those with low and very depressed mood.

The supervisee was able to share their existing strategies and I probed deeply into these to get as much detail as possible. There were pauses where the supervisee would initially say "I don't really know..." but given time and a question such as "What would a person watching you notice you do?" they were able to build a coherent picture of the therapeutic support they offered in these two generalised situations.

I use a single page recording sheet in supervision which is plainly in view of the supervisee. On this I jot down key ideas and it provides a visual mind map of our discussion. On my sheet in this session I noted ideas from our discussion such as 'bearing witness to their pain and distress', 'helping them make a state change – walk and talk outside', 'mirroring matching but matching higher or lower to support their emotional regulation', 'ensuring to establish a plan of reconnection with them so they have this in the days ahead and don't feel so alone', 'being a committed advocate and standing up to poor decisions' and 'they haven't failed, we have failed them'. This last point was from the more macro conversation we circled back to about how to view mental health difficulties differently and what the supervisee's organisation could do at wider levels to offer different thinking into this space.

I observed how each day they walked into uncertainty and asking them how they managed to do this. They shared that their workdays were so unpredictable that they had come to be tolerant of ending each day with something unfinished and how this was ok. They named 'It's having grace with yourself' which I said was a beautiful concept and a great one to hold in these types of situations. Their mood was brighter and energised when they left; the process of naming what they do, the knowledge they made more conscious, and some thoughts to continue to build this, had re-anchored them to their strengths and points of control and influence.

Surfacing, reinforcing and reconnecting a supervisee to existing strengths and practice knowledge confirms my view that supervision is like a base camp, essentially a place that where we can rest, reflect, replenish, and get our equipment (and perhaps add to this) in good working order before we head back out to climb the next mountain. If we cannot easily change the stressor, we can change how we respond and continue to strive for new ways and approaches. The therapeutic function of supervision anchors people to existing competencies and capacities and invites them to build these further in flexible and manageable ways.

Moving forward

The final stage of the experiential learning cycle is active experimentation where learning is identified, knowledge gained, and future ways are determined where this can be applied. When I worked in health leadership, we were taught that when people experience disappointment in the health system, namely through a mistake or error, that part of making amends was for the health professionals to identify what learning had taken place and how this would be put into action. This recognised that while the mistake could not be rectified as it had already occurred, it would contribute into positive change for others in the future. This helps a person feel that their experience had meaning and while negative for them, would contribute to better outcomes for others. From here, people feel more able to move forward from the experience, with a sense of repair of it that helped them integrate it.

In assisting a supervisee to develop a coherent narrative, the active experimentation/application step of the cycle helps give meaning to what has been experienced and explored. This might be through confirming existing thinking or adding value to the person's practice or development. When a supervisee is able to articulate what the experience has meant, shown, or taught them, they will more likely move on from it. This contributes to both restoring and strengthening. Questions such as "What if anything might you do differently?" or "What has this reinforced or affirmed for you?" or "If this issue arose next week who do you think you would approach or respond to it in light of your reflection today?" all assist a supervisee to move into the 'letting come' side of the "U' theory where new or reinforced learning can occur. The supervisor can also reinforce key ideas or reflections from the session and ask how the supervisee might put these into action going forward.

Developing a coherent narrative in supervision invites gathering the telling, reflection and making sense of the experience, and then takes one further step in recognition that supervision holds a commitment to ongoing learning. This last step of identifying learning, knowledge and future action provides a form of closure, much like those in the health setting who have a negative experience. Essentially it gives it meaning and a wider context that can be applied further. It brings the experience to a close, allowing it to be put down or let go. This helps prevent against rumination by the supervisee feeling that they have to keep returning to it in an attempt to try and resolve or fix it. Once the learning is identified I often sense relief in my supervisees, and at this point I invite them to gently put the experience down and not let it continue to dominate. They have told their story, explored it deeply, made sense of it, restored from it, and by identifying and taking learning from it, are able to move forward.

The development of a coherent narrative may also lay a future pathway for possible Post Traumatic Growth (PTG). PTG is a concept defined by Calhoun and Tedeschi (2004) as positive personal transformation that occurs in the aftermath of trauma and highly challenging events. They note there are five aspects to this:

1 A sense of new opportunities.
2 Changed or enhanced relationships with others (relating to others).
3 Increased sense of own personal strength
4 A greater appreciation for life in general.
5 Deepening or changes to spiritual or personal belief systems
(Calhoun & Tedeschi, 2004, p. 95)

Tedeschi et al. comment:

Mindful attention to the cognitive, emotional, and interoceptive aftermath of traumatic experience allows one the opportunity, even if just for a moment, to step back and decentre from the experience, thus providing space for perspective taking and potential reappraisal processes.

(Tedeschi, Blevins & Cara, 2015, p. 374)

PTG theory reminds us to look for areas of growth or changes in thinking in supervisees from having worked through challenge and difficulty. Sharing our observations can be very validating and supportive and contributes to a positive sense of self-worth. We do need to take care though that a supervisee has had enough time to express their negative feelings and responses, and to have told their story fully for integration to have occurred before we move to this type of exploration. Rushing a supervisee to try and see positive benefit when they are not ready to, may convey that we do not wish to hear any more about the negative experience anymore and are trying to move them along.

Summary

Without the opportunity to develop a coherent narrative about our experiences, especially those which contain high emotional content, they may continue to intrude in our thoughts, inviting a range of emotions along with them. We all need the opportunity to tell and make sense of events and issues that are affecting us. A supervisor provides a safe space for this telling, and offers back objective questions and observations that help coherence to emerge and learning to be identified. A coherent narrative is an integration of experience and a key role of the therapeutic function of supervision is to enable this when distress is present. Then, when the telling and reflection is complete, critical reflection takes it one step further into learning and the contribution to their professional knowledge and development.

References

Bond, M., & Holland, S. (2011). *Skills of clinical supervision for nurses: A practical guide for supervisees, clinical supervisors and managers.* Berkshire: McGraw-Hill Education.

Calhoun, L. G., & Tedeschi, R. G. (2004). The foundations of posttraumatic growth: New considerations. *Psychological Inquiry, 15*(1), 93–102.

Carroll, M. (2009). From mindless to mindful practice: On learning reflection in supervision. *Psychotherapy in Australia, 15*(4), 38–49. https://search-informit-org.ezproxy.auckland.ac.nz/doi/10.3316/informit.672638297253917.

Davys, A. (2001). A reflective learning process for supervision. In E. Beddoe, & J. Worral (Eds.), *Supervision from rhetoric to reality* (pp. 87–98). Auckland: Auckland College of Education.

Davys, A., & Beddoe, L. (2021). *Best practice in professional supervision: A guide for the helping professions.* 2nd Edition. London: Jessica Kingsley Publishers.

Hawkins, P., & Shohet, R. (2012). *Ebook: Supervision in the helping professions.* Berkshire: McGraw-Hill Education.

Kolb, D. (1984). *Experiential learning as the source of learning and development.* Englewood Cliffs, NJ: Prentice Hall.

Morrison, T. (1993). *Staff supervision in social care.* London: Longman.

Schon, D. (1983). *The reflective practitioner.* New York. Basic books.

Tedeschi, R., Blevins, G., & Cara, L. (2015). From mindfulness to meaning: implications for the theory of posttraumatic growth. *Psychological Inquiry, 26*(4), 373–376.

Thorpe, K. (2004). Reflective learning journals: From concept to practice. *Reflective Practice, 5*(3), 327–343.

Watkins, C. E., Callahan, J. L., & Vîşcu, L. (2019). The common process of supervision process: The Supervision Session Pyramid as a teaching tool in the beginning supervision seminar. *Journal of Contemporary Psychotherapy.* DOI: 10.1007/s10879-019-09436-5.

4   Working with emotions

The therapeutic function of supervision consciously attends to the emotions inherent in human service work. By having the opportunity to process our emotions, we can move to cognitive understanding, and restoring and strengthening naturally follow. In turn, working intentionally with emotions helps address the indirect trauma impacts of the work and supports reducing emotional labour, stress, and distress.

Emotions are a fundamental source of information and knowledge, providing a way so that we can make sense of situations and events. They help us prioritise where to direct our attention and give us motivation to act (Ingham, 2021). Emotions may influence and guide our interactions with others and require analysis as to why we might have responded in a particular way. As a supervisor it is helpful to have a range of ways to support exploring and managing of emotions so that the supervisee can process these and take any learning from them. Supervision can also support in helping with the development of emotional regulation, enabling a supervisee to better manage their emotions in times of challenge, complexity, and uncertainty (Adamson, 2012). In this chapter, a description of emotional containment and understanding of key emotions is provided along with therapeutic ways to work with them.

Supervision as a space for emotional containment

Social service work brings a full spectrum of emotions both in what is encountered in others, and our own response as workers to these. The notion of 'containment' originated for the work of Bion (1959) and has been built on by from Hoshschild's (1983) work on emotional labour. It is further defined by Morrison, Cree, Ruch,

DOI: 10.4324/9781003359036-5

Winter, Hadfield and Hallett (2019) as the ability of an individual to emotionally manage and contain difficult and unbearable feelings in another person, and also the presence of uncertainty. The worker becomes the container for these feelings, while also requiring effort to manage their own responses. Bond and Holland comment that emotional containment requires "expanding your sense of your own personal strength so that you can contain the feelings, psychologically 'holding' that part of you which is feeling emotional and postponing expressing the feelings until a more appropriate time" (Bond & Holland, 2011, p. 150).

The ability to contain helps workers sustain their practice in emotionally charged professional contexts but also requires a safe space to be able to reflect and process their emotional responses such as within supervision. Hawkins and Shohet (2012) note how workers can manage the negative attacks and impacts from clients by being held "within and by the supervisory relationship" (p. 4). The importance of this holding relationship to process emotional responses especially in relation to interactions with clients is also emphasised by Gray, Field, and Brown (2010) who comment:

> An endangered species in this pressured supervisory climate can be the management of emotion...if the emotion of our work is not managed there can be considerable impact on our effectiveness. We don't work well if we are frightened, depressed, grieving or frozen. Expression of negative emotion is crucial in allowing people to come to terms with a situation and move on from it ... supervision must be a place where emotions can be expressed and explored.
>
> (Gray, Field & Brown, 2010, p. 53)

Simply being in contact with people exposes workers to a myriad of life experiences and generates reactions and responses to these. Workers do not arrive in social service work as clean slates without any emotional difficulties or challenges of their own. Carroll (2014) comments

> Supervisees bring strong emotions to supervision: anxiety, embarrassment, shame, fear of failure, worries about being good enough and many others with the supervisor establishing a relationship and environment that provides a 'safe container' for these.
>
> (p. 67)

Turney and Ruch (2018) in their Cognitive Affective Supervisory Approach note the importance of bringing together 'event' information and 'emotion information', (p. 128), where the supervisor acts as the 'container' for these. Ruch (2005) notes that 'such relationships afford practitioners a space where unthinkable experiences can be processed and made thinkable and manageable'.

(p. 675)

The work of emotional containment highlights the application of emotional intelligence where a person perceives, labels, and distinguishes their own and others' emotion, manages and controls their own emotion and impulses, marshals and uses their emotional knowledge to aid in judgement and to develop understanding and relate to others. This enables people to adapt to situations and problem solve in emotionally responsive and competent ways (Goleman, 2004; Weld, 2006; Weld, 2012, p. 58). Ruch (2005) notes that "the linking of feelings and thoughts generates emotional and cognitive development— thoughtfulness—and contributes to the construction of structures for thinking" (p. 662).

Within the context of supervision, a supervisor is also engaged in this type of process, as it is never certain what a supervisee may bring for discussion or arrive in the room with, be it professionally or personally. An agenda item when unpacked may unleash a range of emotions and the supervisor must work to allow for the expression of these, the analysis of them, help the supervisee make meaning from them, and ensure they are processed to the extent that the supervisee can continue on with their work.

The concept of safety in supervision sets the foundation for this emotional exploration to occur. Ingham reports that supervisees who identified their supervision as being a 'safe place' related this to their level of comfort in exploring emotions and/or uncertainties in their work (Ingham, 2021, p. 466). As supervision requires the exposing of practice, it also requires the exposing of the emotions connected to that practice. The commitment to a partnership for learning in supervision gives space for emotional expression and exploration, and indeed welcomes this. The effort of emotional labour and containment can be put down in the supervision space, where it is the supervisor who may find themselves engaged in the management of their own emotions. This again highlights the need for a supervisor to have their own safe space for emotional expression and reflection.

If workers do not have this space to process emotional responses and set down the effort of emotional containment and labour, their emotions and feelings can be suppressed, leading to even more effort to contain them. Cornell (2003) comments:

> You cannot 'get rid' of any of your feelings, no matter how much you may want to, you only send them underground … in exile parts of us become wilder, darker, lonelier, crueler … when they return from exile they are not a pretty sight.
>
> (p. 113)

Suppressed emotions can impact safe practice and take their toll on a person's wellbeing. The supervisor must be in a space where emotions are permittable and seen as valuable sources of emotion to contribute to learning and knowledge. Ingham (2021) summarises the conditions for 'emotionally sensitive supervision' where emotions can be explored:

> Trust, confidentiality, space for containment and uncertainty, explicit agreement and clarity about the nature and focus of supervision, ring fenced and appropriate levels of time and resource allocate to it, an acceptance and awareness of the positive contribution emotional knowledge can give to practice, and value placed on the intersection between personal and professional identities.
>
> (p. 470)

It is in this environment that attention can be given to the range of emotions supervisees (and supervisors) may experience which will now be discussed.

Overwhelm

I had a supervisee present for supervision naming feeling exhausted and identified this as arising from having an unusual number of contacts with people experiencing significant mental health distress. The supervisee had limited time to process these experiences and now found themselves wanting to avoid the workplace, an understandable self-protective response. I asked them to tell me more about what had arisen so I had sufficient context, then I asked them if they could identify the top emotion they were feeling because of this. After a pause they named feeling overwhelmed. I asked them to describe how this felt in them, and what they were noticing in relation to this emotion. They shared that they were waking in the early hours and that their usual restorative actions were not helping. The supervisee presented as flat in mood, a little tearful and tired.

After letting them express their feeling some more, I applied techniques of normalising and validating by naming how bearing witness to the suffering and distress of others can cause us to feel exhausted of empathy. I then invited them to share what they felt they had done well in these interactions as a way of re-anchoring to their capacities and strengths, and they said they felt they had been present, attentive and responsive. They had sought additional help for the people and followed the correct processes. I reinforced this, and I could see their mood lift a little. I then commented that it sounded like not wanting to be at work was an understandable protective response and an attempt to restore themselves. We discussed how emotional impacts can manifest like physical ones, and that just as you would not put a band aid on a sprained ankle, there needs to be an intentional matching of restorative self-care strategies to the intensity of the emotional experience.

This invited a conversation about permission to restore and top up depleted emotional reserves in ourselves. We also talked about how after being the container for suffering, pain, and distress, we need a chance to be able to lift the lid on this and talk through how it was for us, with colleagues and in supervision. My supervisee related to this, saying it is like a mini debrief, and observed how this had happened more naturally in a previous team they were a part of. We talked about how being left with unprocessed emotional experiences can lead these to build up and contribute to the feeling of overwhelm and subsequent exhaustion they were naming. The rest of the session focused on ways for them to consciously and intentionally restore depleted reserves of empathy and energy. I noticed the supervisee began laughing a little and looked less tense and tired. A large part of the reduction in overwhelm for them came from someone holding space for their experiences and reactions and normalising these. By lightening the load of emotionality, they had been carrying and trying to suppress in order to manage, the overwhelm significantly reduced and they felt able to continue with their week.

Disappointment

Gabor Maté in his documentary The Wisdom of Trauma succinctly explains disappointment as sadness. In my experience it could be likened to sadness mixed with frustration. Somewhere in disappointment is a loss of something, perhaps hope, or the belief something would be one way and it is not, and a sense of let-down. Disappointment could be in others, in self, or in something that has not gone as planned, We sense a loss of what could have been and perhaps find ourselves back at a point we did not want to be.

One of my supervisees initially named wanting to express and explore their frustration regarding a work goal not coming together as they hoped. When I invited them to tell me some more about the frustration and what had happened, they identified feeling 'really disappointed' and then began to cry. I quietly let them be with their sadness and then gently acknowledged their being upset and that I could see that what they had been trying to do was very important to them. They agreed and I asked them to tell me about that importance and they shared more about why it mattered. They named that not being able to complete the work goal as they had hoped to, had left feelings of not being able to make a difference in an area that mattered a great deal to them. We talked about that some more and then began exploring what they were already doing and what more they could do. This started to lift their hope again and to reset their goals about what to do next. I was affirming and acknowledging of the great progress that they had made so far and offered a couple of reframes and alternative thoughts and strategies for them to reflect on. The session finished with them naming that they were feeling better and more positive.

Disappointment can be generated by something deeper than just the presenting experience. It may be connected to a greater personal meaning such as a belief or value, even a want, and underneath this, may be a previous life need that was not met. Disappointment can feel overwhelming because of this, with people experiencing a deep let-down that may not even feel rational in the current situation. Or people may know intellectually that their disappointment is out of proportion to the experience but feel powerless to explain why.

A supervisor might ask them to reflect what else might be driving their response, is it something about a value or belief or something from their life experiences as a child or adult? It is here the boundary between offering a therapeutic safe place and engaging in therapy once again emerges. While a supervisee might share that the issue really matters because of something that happened to them in earlier life, the supervisor will certainly acknowledge, validate, and normalise this but not deeply unpack it. If the theme keeps re-surfacing and causing impact in their professional life, it is helpful to invite the supervisee to consider exploring this in counselling or therapy. If a supervisee understands and can name a deep-seated earlier life trigger that fires disappointment, this insight will help them better manage it in the future even simply through the articulation of this. Deeper personal unpacking of it best belongs elsewhere in a more therapy-based space.

Anger

Anger is an emotion that signals a sense of being over controlled in some way, or a perceived reaction to injustice and restriction. It may be a response to a real or perceived threat to both physical and psychological safety. It is linked to the fight aspect of the stress response designed to stop or make a threat go away. A person may feel angry that something is unfair and fails to take into account their view, voice or ideas. Anger is a self-protective emotion, designed to generate energy to take action or to stop other emotions such as shame, sadness, helplessness and powerlessness. It is a very helpful emotion if managed well, as it can bring about change and surface what a person is thinking or feeling. However, if not managed well it can cause regrettable behaviour, and at its worst, rage. The goals of working with anger is that it is expressed safely, assertively communicated, and that people have self-management of it for example through self-calming techniques to reduce escalation in the moment.

I had a supervisee who was feeling very angry about being overlooked in an interaction with a colleague and wanted to talk this through in supervision. I decided to amplify the voice of their anger, allowing it full expression, and invited them to take a piece of paper and a black marker pen, and draw and write as furiously and angrily as they liked on the paper, and to not censor it. Initially they hesitated and then embraced the activity, writing a swear word as hard as they could across the page and pushing their anger and hurt out through the pen and onto the paper. I asked them to tell me what they had really wanted to say in the interaction, and they gave voice to the overlooked feeling and unfairness of it. Deep within this anger they recognised was being overlooked when they were younger. Once their anger was safely expressed through the paper and the uncensored statement, it began to dissipate, and we moved to strategise as to how they could address the unfairness in a calm assertive manner. We rehearsed this until it felt comfortable and by the end of the session we agreed that their anger had now provided an opportunity for them to practise assertive communication.

Irritation can be named instead of anger, possibly because it is seen as more socially acceptable or permissible, yet when explored anger often sits close by. Irritation can develop into anger if not explored and expressed. Irritation may also indicate stress, strain, and fatigue, where the worker cannot easily find their compassion or empathy due to having given out a lot of this, and instinctively needing to self-protect. Exploring the irritation invites expression of either a sense of being over controlled or restricted in some way, the effort of suppressing and inducing emotion, or depleted compassion.

I had a supervisee name that they wanted to talk through feeling irritated by agency rules and administrative tasks that they were finding extremely frustrating especially in meetings. As they shared this, I could see they were digging their fingernails into the palm of their hand, almost in a bid to control or suppress anger. I invited them to tell me more about the irritation, and consciously increased my tone of voice to be more animated and contain more energy rather than be soothing. I gave permission for them to bring the anger forward by normalising statements such as "That sounds totally frustrating!" They became less reserved and said how much it annoyed them and how it felt like such a waste of time. I continued to encourage their expression of this, and they eventually said they felt really angry and frustrated about a number of things and felt they had nowhere to direct this, and that it was not permissible for them to feel like this. They saw their workplace as having an unspoken culture of everyone 'being nice and calm' yet the effort of having to sustain this seemed to be driving up the levels of frustration, a great description of 'surface acting'.

I said that I thought anger was a great emotion and they seemed both surprised and relieved by this. I said that anger tells us we perceive injustice and draws attention to those areas where we might feel overcontrolled or suppressed. I asked what they found helped with anger when we cannot easily change the stressor, and calming techniques were not enough. We talked about the need for physical expression of it through exercise so the tension and adrenaline are released safely. This was difficult in their workday and afterwards due to family commitments, but we discussed taking fifteen minutes to go and walk really hard up the hilly road outside their work, sending all the anger through their feet into the concrete and to push against the hill as they powered up it. They laughed but seemed quite taken with this idea, and when I asked if it felt feasible, they said it did. We also discussed closing their office door and doing a really hard standing press up against the wall, literally pushing all the frustrated energy out into the wall.

We then discussed points of influence and choice they did have in their workplace and how to use these to the best effect to help reduce the irritation and anger. At this point I reduced the energy in my tone of voice to help support calming for when they left the room. After the session as we walked back down the corridor, we giggled together about secretly pressing our feet really strongly into the carpeted floor. Their mood was considerably lighter and relieved, both to have some strategies but also to have validated and given permission to have anger and to express it safely.

Anger can also mask hurt, and I had another supervisee who had felt let-down by their work colleagues and presented as very angry about this in supervision. I invited them to tell me about what had happened and pressed them for detail of this (so helping with the expression and the development of a coherent narrative about it). As they talked it out, I could hear the hurt that was present and I asked them about this, saying "That sounded like it could have been hurtful, was that how it was?" They quickly agreed, and we then talked about the hurt and they identified how this related to some earlier experiences as a child.

I suggested that perhaps the anger was protective as it sought to fight back in this adult context against the early experiences of being hurt, unseen, and dismissed. I then invited them to consider what might have been happening for the other people in the interaction, so assisting them to reframe it. They were able to articulate what might have happened for the other people and how what had happened toward them was likely not deliberate or personal. We managed to have a laugh which helped dissipate the anger further and continued to defuse it as they gained a different perspective. We then discussed what they might do a little differently in the future in terms of their response, and they were able to name some good strategies here and I affirmed their timeout strategy they had chosen at the time.

Another supervisee identified a mixture of anger and frustration resulting in reactivity in a range of situations. I noticed while they were furiously talking and their anger escalating, that I was slowing and deepening my breath almost in a bid to help them calm. I decided to share this observation of my own response, saying I felt like I wanted them to breath with me. The person paused and we took a moment to slow our breathing together, essentially engaged in a process of co-regulation. They were then able to recognise older triggers which we identified were heightening their stress arousal response.

We then talked about the increased cortisol levels they were likely experiencing and how taking a minute per hour to consciously focus on breath when they were feeling heightened would help reduce this. I suggested for that minute they try doing a two second pause before exhaling, doing a longer exhale, and counting two seconds before breathing in again. I also invited them to be curious about what was happening, so their reaction and that of others to create a conscious pause between reacting and responding. In professional situations the ability to calm and self-manage anger can get people through to a safer place where it is ok to express and name the anger.

Shame

Possibly one of the most debilitating emotions we can experience is shame. Dolezal and Gibson (2022) note that shame is a "negative self-conscious emotion" (p. 3) that carries fear and worry about how other people perceive us. Often installed in at an early age, and heightened through experiences of abuse and neglect, persistent shaming can turn hurtful experiences inward to become messages of being unlikable, unlovable, and this generates feelings of loss of belonging and acceptance. Children being concrete egocentric thinkers will tend to make sense of abusive behaviour from adults as evidence that they, not the adult's behaviour, are wrong or flawed in some way. Roland Summit's sexual abuse accommodation syndrome (1983) shows the process a child moves through when experiencing sexual abuse including stages of secrecy, helplessness, entrapment and accommodating, delayed disclosure and retraction. Underneath all of these stages, and applicable to all forms of abuse and neglect, is the likely development of shame which contributes to feelings of being alone, unseen and perceived as not worthy of love and care.

Dolezal and Gibson (2022) note that these early relational experiences can contribute to a persistent "shame anxiety" about being "judged, labelled, or rejected" by others (p. 4). Relational trauma, especially in childhood, sets the conditions for a high propensity to shame, and as supervisors, if we are aware of a supervisee having a history of relational trauma, this will alert us to this possible propensity. Dolezal and Gibson (2022) observe that shame is a key feature of many of the maladaptive behaviours that may follow a traumatic experience (p. 5). The emotion of shame is so strong that people will often go to great lengths to avoid the intense discomfort of it. While guilt can draw our attention to a wrong we may have done and can learn from, shame does not serve much purpose except to show a desire for belonging and acceptance, and may indicate a number of highly negative internalised messages.

In a supervisee we might see shame evidenced by high levels of apology for self, immobilisation and avoidance of certain situations, heightened sensitivity, fear of loss of belonging and connection, intense self-critique including high levels of self-admonishment, embarrassment, and feelings of inadequacy. Persistent rumination may also indicate a returning to an experience that shame has become linked to. There may also be defensive levels of anger as the supervisee attempts to push back or protect against the possibility of shame, or avoidance of relational situations that may carry a risk of self-exposure where the perceived flawed self would become seen and potentially rejected again.

Working with shame in a therapeutic way in supervision requires kindness and sensitivity, which can in turn, help a supervisee learn to direct these responses toward themselves. Dolezal and Gibson (2022) suggest having 'shame sensitivity' in human service and relational based work, which equally applies to the supervision context. They observe shame sensitivity to contain three key areas: acknowledging shame, avoiding shaming, and addressing shame (Dolezal & Gibson, 2022). These include having an understanding of shame and naming and recognising shame in organisational contexts, sensitivity and awareness of the possibility of shame in interpersonal interactions and understanding how a person experiences shame and developing self-compassionate responses instead. As supervisors our overall intention is to ensure that the relationship remains intact and can be deepened by sensitive exploration into the vulnerability of shame. The underlying fear of rejection or exclusion that is the core of shame will therefore not be experienced.

Shame sensitivity in supervision includes careful attention to the giving of feedback. Carroll (2011) notes that shame out of all of the emotions is the one that most impedes and blocks learning (p. 18). The giving of feedback where the supervisor is aware of the supervisee being sensitive to shame, relies on a warm accepting relationship where, for example, the supervisor can show vulnerability in briefly sharing their own mistakes to help normalise experiences which reduces a sense of isolation. This can help reassure a supervisee and lift them more quickly out of a place of shame. It helps to focus on an area of learning very specifically, and in no way constructing this as a form of personal failing. Careful and conscious attention to our use of language is imperative to this. I liken working with shame to a walking in a field of fragile flowers so taking great care as to where I place my feet. In supervision this metaphor translates to the words I chose and where I place them.

While we must address areas of practice that are contributing to wider impacts, it is important that we address these in a way that maintains relationship, as shame can cause withdrawal from supervision. We need to be able to reinforce positive qualities of the supervisee, share our noticing of what went well amidst something that went wrong, and remind a supervisee of what we enjoy and appreciate about them. This reduces the fear of not belonging by instead maintaining connection and relationship. We can invite them to practise self-compassion and self-kindness which can reduce shame and strengthen psychological wellbeing over time.

I had a supervisee who despite having appearances of upbeat and easy going had a high propensity to shame linked to childhood experiences. This presented in their fear of processes such as performance appraisals which they would go to great lengths to avoid for fear of hearing negative feedback. On one occasion they came to supervision bursting with pride about how they had applied a new assessment tool and what they had then done. Unfortunately, there was a serious omission in the following intervention for two very vulnerable people and as part of attending to practice safety, I knew I had to address this. I acknowledged the great work they had done in the first part of their work and then gently said I was wondering about the two vulnerable people.

Before I could say any more their eyes widened and their hand flew to their mouth in horror as they realised their error. Shame quickly set in as they berated themselves severely about the omission fuelled further by it now being witnessed by me. I gently said it was just a mistake, and that given we could not change what had happened, we could do something now and invited them to tell me about what they could do to attend to this. From here we worked out a plan. I then reassured them that they had done a great job at the beginning, and this was a learning moment which they had immediately taken up. I also asked them to be kind to themselves about making a mistake as we all do. I thanked them for being vulnerable and looking at this with me. While their fire of shame continued to burn a little, it was not as intense, and the session ended on a positive note. Carroll (2014) calls these critical moments in supervision, which require compassionate, kind, and courageous engagement, ultimately strengthening the supervisory relationship.

Anxiety

There is a noticeable increase in anxiety among younger workers, and placed within the Aotearoa, New Zealand context, this is hardly surprising given they have grown up within the context of the Canterbury earthquakes, a terrorist attack, and a pandemic. The COVID-19 pandemic and other global events such as climate change have introduced a persistent hum of anxiety into people's lives. It is likely this affects some younger people more who may have had accumulated less adverse life experiences to build resilience to manage this. Add the pressures of modern living such as negative social media impacts, worry about housing and income, and the inherent uncertainty and complexity present in social service work due to the unpredictability of human behaviour, and it is hardly surprising anxiety surfaces within the context of supervision.

Anxiety like all emotions is a cyclic response of body and thoughts and can be highly distressing. It can activate the freeze and flight aspect of the stress response, leading to inaction and a failure to respond in work situations. Because it is a combination of a nervous system response which is body based, body work can be an effective way to respond to it, such as grounding, vagal nerve exercises, and breath work.

The cognitive process of anxiety is often anticipatory, so trying to manage uncertainty by problem solving which quickly can become stress and worry. Frazier et al. (2011) make the point that trying to control events into the future can often be distressing and lead to hypervigilance and anxiety. Anxiety can also stem from rumination through trying to problem solve events already passed by bringing them back to mind. As the stress response is activated with anxiety, the body consequences of this can be very severe namely through panic. In a panic attack there is increased heart rate, sweating, terror and shaking.

There are ways to manage and counter anxiety, but it is important to recognise that individual anxiety responses are person specific, and that time is taken to enquire and understand how the anxiety is being experienced by the supervisee and then identify with them what might best support reducing this. A supervisor needs to begin with exploring and supporting the development of understanding of the supervisee's anxiety, and the following questions can assist with that.

1 How do you know when you are anxious? What is happening in your body? What thoughts are you having? What else is happening?
2 Imagine understanding anxiety as peeling back layers of an onion. Think of a situation that you felt anxious about and keep peeling it back, layer by layer until you identify what the true cause of the anxiety is. Speak this out loud to yourself.

3 Are there any older childhood messages or experiences you can track your anxiety back to?
4 What do you typically do when you feel anxious?
5 What is the most helpful way you have found to manage anxiety?

(Weld, 2017)

In human service work there is an exchange of energy. If our energy is stressed, anxious or depressed, there could be serious consequences for those with whom we are working. Anxiety is an emotion that, left unmanaged and unexplored, can contribute to mistakes in our work and professional dangerousness. However, it can also be a rich place of learning and contribute to an opening up of discussion and awareness for other people to increase their safety and wellbeing.

I met with a supervisee via remote means during a lockdown response to a COVID-19 outbreak, who identified having a strong bodily response to facing work each day, and realised this was becoming overwhelming to the point of debilitating. We identified that their work did not usually prompt this response when they were in the office, and that they had also been working primarily from their bedroom due to being in a shared living situation. The natural boundary between work and home had become disrupted with their usual morning routine of not looking at work communication until on the way to work changed by waking up and looking at emails in bed. Their usual safe sanctuary of their bedroom had now been intruded upon by their work.

I explored what helped their physiological symptoms to abate and they were able to name practical strategies that assisted with this. I commended and reinforced these strategies and encouraged them to not look at work in their bed. They also recognised they had lost daily structure, and that going for a daily walk greatly helped the symptoms the next day. They recognised how they had dropped off from social connection with friends and family and that this likely was not helping.

As it was not their actual work causing the response, we explored other factors exacerbated by the lockdown. These revealed a very future focus on trying to manage and achieve mastery of three personal key issues not within their control. They revealed how much thinking time they gave to these issues and how they were constantly trying to problem solve and resolve them as a way to manage uncertainty. We talked about this and explored points of certainty in their lives, what was within their control and what was not. We also discussed how to notice thoughts and check if they were serving them well, and to limit the time given to specific areas of concern in their life. As Eckhart Tolle's (2001) work exemplifies, we are ultimately in charge of how we think about what enters our minds or what we bring to mind. This can help leverage some control in thinking patterns which feel out of control. Our minds are tools, and we can reassert control over how we apply them.

Anxiety can also be helped by remaining more present through both body grounding, namely attending to the vagal nerve and overall nervous system so activating the parasympathetic nervous system (this will be discussed further in Chapter 8), sensory noticing, and breath work. Bringing focused attention through doing something quite different for ten minutes, or watching a show or reading is another helpful way to interrupt a potential looping of thoughts. Committing to finishing a task can also help bring focus back to the present and stops the mind and energy being pulled to this. Turning and facing what needs to be done can reduce anxiety, although doing this may require courage which will be explored in Chapter 7. Overall noticing the thoughts, asking if they are helpful and being curious about them without joining with them, helps to locate the mind as a tool and one we can use to best serve us.

Supervision is an ideal place to explore anxiety as often the simple tasking of naming fear, worry and uncertainty can help reduce the impact of it, especially if a plan is developed to move forward. Engaging in small immediate steps establishes points of control and certainty, and the ability to continue to emotionally recognise and adapt to what may not be resolvable. Anxiety can be exhausting and just like other forms of stress, the body needs to be able to express the adrenaline and cortisol that has been activated. Exercise is a great way to do this, as is being out in fresh air and interacting (safely in a pandemic!) with others. Exercise also helps with sleep, as lack of sleep can reduce the ability to cognitively manage difficulties. In supervision we can enquire how a person is sleeping and explore any behavioural and environmental barriers to this. Reducing stimuli before bed is key so the mind is not unduly activated. During times of widespread stress, it helps to reduce exposure to this such as following constant news reports which can trigger an activated stress response.

It is also important for us to check on our overall wellbeing and reduce stimulants such as caffeine and sugar which can cause the body to feel jittery and mirror the feelings of anxiety. People can be in habit of coffee in the morning to get going, and a fix of sugar around mid-afternoon to keep going. Unfortunately, too much coffee speeds up the heart rate sometimes causing increased cortisol, and sugar gives a temporary surge of pleasure and energy, but this can quickly dissipate, lowering mood and can impact inflammatory conditions.

Having structure to one's day, recognising what is and what is not within our control, noticing our thoughts and not joining with these, instead checking their accuracy and building tolerance of them so they are supportive and not generating emotional suffering are all helpful strategies. Grounding and anchoring through feet placed firmly on the ground, very intentionally using all five senses to bring awareness to the present and saying 'nothing bad is happening right now' can help reduce panic, followed by gently bringing focus to the breath and simply allowing the 2 second pause during inhaling and exhaling through the nose (with a deliberate longer exhale), can soothe the central nervous system. Developing a daily wellbeing plan can help achieve mastery over anxiety, and this will be explored further in Chapter 8. Replacing a focus on worry with one of gratitude or intentionally noticing what is ok and what can be appreciated can also shift and reset a mind primed to notice what is wrong or worrying to one that sees good and positive aspects of life.

I checked back the next day with the supervisee who was experiencing high physiological distress and thanked them for what they shared and acknowledged their self-awareness. I gently reinforced some of the strategies we discussed and offered the possibility of bringing our next session forward if this would be of help which they did. I also suggested that if their symptoms worsened that contacting their health clinic and doctor would be a supportive strategy. As a supervisor we are part of worker's safety and wellbeing network and while natural occurring social supports are always best, there are times where a slightly more detached and objective support can help people ride the more difficult waves in their lives. Knowing we are not alone is itself very therapeutic.

Grief

Loss is inevitable in life and grief provides a way for us to process what is now different and adapt to this. Because it is inevitable, it is likely most supervisees will experience this at some stage. This could be the loss of a relationship, a loved one, changes in life such as children leaving home, or the loss of a hope or aspiration. The challenge of personal loss while holding a professional role requires attention to how to best manage grief as a requirement of our working lives. Grieving is the expression of an emotional wound, and like a physical wound, we need to give it time and attention to heal (Weld, 2017).

The therapeutic function of supervision provides this space to support the expression of grief and can assist to recognise and integrate the loss that is being experienced.

While it can be helpful to understand that grief responses such as denial and anger are a normal and understandable way of trying to process a significant change or loss; it can be unhelpful to suggest that people move through these responses in a staged or sequential manner. Everyone has their own way of adapting and responding to loss and there is not a prescribed or 'correct' way to do this (Weld, 2017). Overall, it is better to come from a place of 'not knowing' rather than presuming understanding (Neimeyer, 1999, p. 68) when working with a supervisee who is grieving. We do not know this person's unique experience and relationship to what has been lost, and while theoretical knowledge is helpful, we need to determine how it may support this person and their situation.

If a supervisee experiences the loss of a person, the attachment to them and the role they had in life will give insight into the possible impact this will be having (Longaker, 1997). We can support a supervisee who has experienced loss to both immerse themselves in their grief and reorientate to the present by practical tasks that provide respite from the pain of active grieving (Neimeyer, 2000). Neimyer also suggests that grieving becomes complicated if a person either becomes located in solely feeling or immersed in doing to the exclusion of the other, it may be experienced as "getting stuck in relentless rumination or prolonged avoidance of the pain" (p. 43). We can encourage a supervisee to go with the waves of grief as they roll in, rather than suppress or avoid them and normalise crying, sobbing, yelling, and wailing as healthy expressions of grief and useful ways to help to release feelings and upset. I also suggest people make sure they take time, go gently with themselves, and allow space for their grief rather than rush headlong back into work life. This is also applicable to the loss of a dearly loved pet who was a cherished member of their family.

We can also suggest exercise, relaxation, or everyday 'normal' everyday activities to help manage stress and re-engage with life. Neimeyer talks about the grieving process moving between "feeling and doing" (Neimeyer, 2000, p. 43). He comments that in opening ourselves to grief we can run the risk of "focusing relentlessly on the pain of loss, which can be a bit like staring unblinkingly into the sun – it may actually be damaging if our gaze is sustained too long" (Neimeyer, 2000, p. 42). Instead, he suggests that people use periods of mourning to attend to feelings of loss, and then reorient to the physical tasks of home and life (Neimeyer, 2000, p. 43).

Talking and writing about the memories of who the person was and what they were like can help to keep them present and validated. When a supervisee shared the loss of their father with me, I asked them to tell me his name and then invited them to describe to me what he was like. We sat quietly, her talking, me listening and learning about him, as she brought him back into the world through her memories and experiences.

As grief helps us transition from the physical to a spiritual relationship, (Neimeyer, 2000) we might still 'talk' to the person and share important events with them in some way. Symbolic connection to the person, also helps, such as keeping an item of their clothing, putting up photos, or having special things around that were significant to the person. It might be jewellery that when worn brings the person into closer connection with someone that has gone. These objects might be placed in full view somewhere in the home where they can have specific symbolic meaning and help hold the person in someone's life despite them no longer being physically there. All of these symbolic acts can help people to embrace someone's memory and help to establish the spiritual relationship to the person.

Loss and change, especially through events that are sudden and traumatic, can seriously impact and challenge people's beliefs and views of the world. A supervisee may find that their existing spiritual beliefs are not sufficiently sustaining and question them instead. Trying to make meaning of abrupt, sudden, or prolonged loss can be extremely difficult. For some people, finding meaning may not be the key objective; instead, it might be to make meaning of the person's contribution to life, or of the situation that has changed (Weld, 2017). Meaning may also come from the recognition and celebration of how a person contributed to loved ones and their lives. Neimeyer (1999) calls this an 'imprint' and suggests that, especially when someone dies, we can recognise and see how they contributed to us. This might be the passing on of a love of nature, a sense of loyalty, a belief in fairness or a trait such as an ability to see something in a quirky or funny way.

Sometimes a range of factors, including multiple losses in a short timeframe, or a traumatic sudden loss, can create a prolonged complex grieving process. This may become evident if a supervisee is unable to take part and enjoy normal activities and resume responsibilities in their lives, or are engaging in harmful activities, such as substance abuse as a form of coping. They may also be reactive, with persistent feelings of bitterness, guilt, loss of trust, rage and blame directed at others or themselves. They could be experiencing disrupted sleep patterns, increased anxiety, low mood and depression. A supervisee may also be experiencing complex grief if there is no noticeable change in their level of distress and they appear 'consumed' or solely focused on what has been lost. For supervisees with indications of complex grief, therapeutic support within supervision is likely not enough, and the supervisor can encourage and support them to access targeted therapies including trauma counselling that can help them manage their loss.

Summary

Working with the cross section of emotions that supervisees will experience in their work and share in supervision is a core feature of the therapeutic function of supervision. A deliberate focus and enquiry into emotional responses can help workers process and make sense of them. Increased self-awareness of emotions and their management contribute greater emotional knowledge which can be applied back to the workplace. Staying emotionally safe and well in our work supports overall mental and psychological wellbeing which deserves the same attention we bring to our physical wellbeing. Working emotionally also requires the supervisor to be conscious of and attending to their own emotional state especially when providing a container for the emotional expression of others. A failure to do this will likely contribute to the supervisor being less emotionally open and even avoid emotional discussion for fear of being triggered or activated personally. This is another important reminder of the energy exchange that occurs in supervision and that the supervisor's own supervision is of an equally reflective and therapeutic nature.

References

Adamson, C. (2012). Supervision is not politically innocent. *Australian Social Work, 65*(2), 185–196. DOI: 10.1080/0312407X.2011.618544.

Bion, W (1959). Attacks on linking. *International Journal of Psychoanalysis, 40*, 308–315.

Bond, M., & Holland, S. (2011). *Skills of clinical supervision for nurses: A practical guide for supervisees, clinical supervisors and managers.* Berkshire: McGraw-Hill Education.

Carroll, M. (2011). Supervision: A journey of lifelong learning. In R. Shohet (Ed.), *Supervision as transformation: A passion for learning* (pp. 14–28). London: Jessica Kingsley Publishers.

Carroll, M. (2014). *Effective supervision for the helping professions.* London: SAGE Publications.

Cornell, A.W. (2003). *The radical acceptance of everything – Living a focusing life.* Berkeley, CA: Calluna Press.

Dolezal, L., & Gibson, M. (2022). Beyond a trauma-informed approach and towards shame-sensitive practice. *Humanities and Social Sciences Communications, 9*, 214. DOI: 10.1057/S41599-022-01227-Z.

Frazier, P., Keenan, N., Anders, S., Perera, S., Shallcross, S., & Hintz, S. (2011). Perceived past, present, and future control and adjustment to stressful life events. *Journal of Personality and Social Psychology, 100*(4), 749–765.

Goleman, D. (2004). *Emotional intelligence and working with emotional intelligence.* London. Bloomsbury.

Gray, I., Field, R., & Brown. K. (2010). *Effective leadership, management and supervision in health and social care.* Exeter: Learning Matters.

Ingham, R. (2021). Emotionally sensitive supervision. In K. O'Donoghue, & L. Engelbrecht (Eds.), *The Routledge international handbook of social work supervision* (pp. 462–471). London: Routledge International.

Hawkins, P., & Shohet, R. (2012). *Ebook: Supervision in the helping professions.* Berkshire: McGraw-Hill Education.

Hocshschild, A. R. (1983). *The managed heart.* Berkeley: University of California Press.

Longaker, C. (1997). *Facing death and facing hope.* New York: Broadway Books.

Morrison, F., Cree, V., Ruch, G., Winter, K., Hadfield, M., & Hallett, S. (2019). Containment - Exploring the concept of agency in children's statutory encounters with social workers. *Childhood, 26*(1), 98–112. ISSN 0907-5682.

Neimeyer, R. (1999). Narrative strategies in grief therapy. *Journal of Constructivist Psychology, 12*, 65–85.

Neimeyer, R. (2000). *Lessons of loss: A guide to coping.* Victoria: Australian Centre for Grief and Bereavement.

Ruch, G. (2005). Reflective practice in contemporary child care social work: The role of containment. *British Journal of Social Work, 37*(4), 659–680.

Summit, R. (1983). The child sexual abuse accommodation syndrome. *Child abuse and Neglect, 7*(2), 177–193.

Tolle, E. (2001). *The power of now.* London: Hodder and Stoughton.

Turney, D., & Ruch, G. (2018). What makes it so hard to look and to listen? Exploring the use of the cognitive and affective supervisory approach with children's social work managers. *Journal of Social Work Practice, 32*(2), 125–138. DOI: 10.1080/02650533.2018.1439460.

Weld, N. (2006). Awareness and emotions. Social work now. *The Practice Journal of Child, Youth and Family, 35*, 4–7.

Weld, N. (2012). *A practical guide to transformative supervision for the helping professions.* London: Jessica Kingsley Publishing.

Weld, N. (2017). *E Ko te Matakahi Maire therapeutic social work.* Stand Children Services. Wellington: Tū Māia.

5   Working with relational dynamics

Providing a therapeutic function in supervision requires attending to relational dynamics, both ours and the supervisee's. Human relationships can generate great satisfaction and joy, and also difficulties, stress and distress for supervisees, be this with service users, colleagues, or people within their wider professional network. As the core of human service work is with people, our views, attitudes, assumptions, and beliefs are regularly tested and challenged. Schamess (2006) notes that "at best supervision increases supervisees' understanding of unconscious meaning, promotes empathy, improves clinical skills, enhances ego functioning, and expands relational capacity" (p. 428). Powerful learning happens within the context of relationship, and supervision offers an ideal place to explore and reflect on the interactions, responses, and behaviour within these, especially when causing emotional impacts. This enhances the conscious use of self in our work and acknowledges the value and importance of the interdependent nature of what we do.

Personality, beliefs, and values

Conversations about relational dynamics reveal values, beliefs, attitudes, and how we consciously bring ourselves to the work we do. When we are working with people, we bring both our professional self and the personal self to the professional relationship and need to critically reflect on the balance of these. Too little of our personal self can make us appear cold or distant, resulting in people struggling to connect to us, while too much may result in confusion for people who might view us a friend, and hence the goals and boundaries of the work become unclear (Weld, 2008, 2017).

DOI: 10.4324/9781003359036-6

Our personal self is shaped by our family, culture, values, education, experiences, relationships, and socioeconomic class (Connolly & Harms, 2009, p. 8). The intersection of this with our professional self (informed by our training, ethics and standards, code of conduct, colleagues, agency culture, supervision, and previous practice experiences) influences the type of practitioner and supervisor we become (Connolly & Harms, 2009, p. 8). Professional supervision acknowledges these two selves and commits to exploring both within the context of quality service delivery.

Dewane (2006, p. 544) comments that "melding the professional self of what one knows (training, knowledge, techniques) with the personal self of who one is (personality traits, belief systems and life experience) is a hallmark of skilled practice". She suggests that we operationalise our self in our work through our personality, belief systems, relational dynamics, examining our anxiety, and how we use self-disclosure.

Through conscious use of our personality, we bring aspects of ourselves that help people to make a connection with us and support the relational nature of social service work (Edwards & Bess, 1998; Dewane, 2006). This might include traits such as humour, warmth, reliability, kindness, and the way we approach life in general. Our beliefs and values are initially shaped through the process of our socialisation and can contain important threads intrinsically woven by significant people in our lives, especially when we were children. Our belief system informs how we view the world, including what we value and how we respond to challenge and difficulty. Edwards and Bess (1998, p. 98) comment:

> In this is the requirement to uncover an understanding of the personal solutions to lifelong dilemmas created by childhood crises and traumas which have created the 'unconscious ordering principles' (Atwood & Stolorow, 1993, p. 181) that the therapist relies on to understand life experiences as these will affect the approach and direction the therapist will take. Conscious knowledge of these helps a therapist to use them constructively while not knowing of them could be counterproductive.

These 'unconscious ordering principles' may be part of the 'blind' or 'hidden' aspects of the JoHari window and may predict how we approach different situations. An example of this would be if a person's ordering principles have contributed to an internal or external locus of control, a concept developed by Rotter (1954) to explain the degree of control people feel they have over their lives. An internal locus of control indicates a person believes they can influence events around them whereas an external locus of control is suggestive of person who feels that life events are more likely to be out of their influence and happen to them.

We also need to revisit what brought us into human service work, and indeed even supervising, and be clear about our motivations for this. These might be life experiences that contributed to the development of beliefs or values that we strive to uphold. Early negative experiences can be turned into a determination and dedication to not replicate these as adults, an example being cruelty learnt from childhood abuse not acted on and instead turned to actions of kindness. There may be other personal drivers such as a desire to be liked or needed or to be seen to have worth if this was not experienced as a child.

Hawkins and Shohet (2012) acknowledge the presence of 'shadow motives' so those which we may speak less about or have less awareness of such as early experiences of personal powerlessness leading to an over exertion of power. It is important these are in a place of resolution, so they do not dominate our actions, potentially leading to professionally dangerous behaviour. Attempting to heal ourselves through work with people struggling with vulnerability creates risk for both them and us. Supervision is an ideal place to examine and reflect on beliefs, motivations, and values and check if these are still serving us well, and also to identify if further action is required to address our own past hurts.

These questions from the work of Dewane (2006) and Edwards and Bess (1998) can be helpful to explore our beliefs, values and ordering principles in supervision, and as a personal reflection:

1 What is my view of how the world works?
2 What traumas or life crises have shaped my world-view?
3 What are my top three personal beliefs or values?
4 If someone has a very different belief system from my own, how do I work with this?
5 What would I say motivates me to do this type of work?
6 What are the top three attributes and skills I think I bring to it?
7 What do I enjoy about the work?
8 What triggers my flight/fight response or makes uncomfortable about my work?
9 What need is doing this work fulfilling in me?

(Edwards & Bess, 1998; Dewane, 2006, p. 550)

We can be protective of our core beliefs and values as these likely come from early experiences that have shaped our sense of identity. To therefore examine or challenge these can feel vulnerable or even a betrayal of ourself or others in our lives. Supervision is a good place to develop a reframe of a belief, value or motivation that is perhaps no longer serving someone well, and to let it go while appreciating the role it played at a different stage of our life. It is important there is congruence between our values, beliefs and the work we are engaged in as incongruence can lead to personal dissonance and heightened emotional labour to act in ways we fundamentally do not believe in or value.

The use of self-disclosure

Within the supervision context, there is freer exchange of self-disclosure than would be observed in a client worker relationship. The use of self-disclosure supports relationships but only in an intentional and well managed way. Dewane (2006, p. 544) comments, "Self-disclosure must lead to growth; it should deepen the capacity for insight and for relationship. In other words, it should be for furthering the therapeutic alliance. It is ultimately predetermined for the client's benefit". This is a useful self-check to ensure self-disclosure in both supervision and practice is meeting a need of the person and not ourselves.

In the getting to know each stage of developing the supervisor relationship, sharing some personal information helps build engagement, rapport and connection. This might be as simple as sharing where we grew up and who we live with. Self-disclosure may continue now and then when relevant and intended to contribute to the supervisee's personal and professional learning and development. In both supervision and practice, self-disclosure is not useful when it takes the focus away from the supervisee or client, causing a shift in the support dynamic, a drop in credibility, or closing communication down. Even in the early stages of developing the supervisory relationship, we should be asking ourselves why we are sharing this information when we self-disclose, and be clear of our motivation for this.

Self-disclosure can be helpful to support development if done as a personal observation in relation to what is being shared in supervision to both convey understanding and invite further reflection, such as "I found myself tense up as you shared how she spoke to you , is that how you felt?" It can also help a supervisee experience normalisation and validation in their response if the supervisor shares an understanding of this.

Here are three questions adapted from Dewane (2006) to consider before using self-disclosure:

1 Is this disclosure for the person's benefit or is it for a possibly unnamed need/benefit of my own?
2 How will this disclosure support the person?
3 Is there another way I could contribute to this person's work that doesn't require direct personal sharing of my own experience?

The utilisation of self in undertaking the therapeutic function in supervision requires honesty, self-awareness, a commitment to professional and personal development, and careful attention to what is happening in and around us.

Counter-transference and parallel process

The concepts of transference, counter-transference and parallel process provide a unique opportunity to both build self-awareness and alleviate stress and distress in relational interactions. Essentially within types of transference, there is some degree of unconscious projection of feelings, thoughts, and behaviours often related to previous life experiences (Schamess, 2006). Sudbery (2002) comments that "Deeper relational work requires greater use of self, which in turn raises the possibility of transference and countertransference being present" (p. 154). It is useful to have good awareness of these concepts and be able to apply them in supervision to help support the therapeutic function, along with the development of understanding and self-knowledge. Schamess (2006) notes that "when supervisors reflect on transferential themes they listen differently and understand more fully what supervisees tell them. Consequentially, supervisees relate more empathetically to patients and also to significant others" (p. 432).

Counter-transference is when a worker transfers feelings and responses arising from one experience onto a current situation with a service user. An example would be a service user who reminds the supervisee of a person in their own life, be this positive or negative. The worker may view the person through the lens of understanding they adopted for this prior relationship and project this onto the person. If the experience was a negative one, they may self-protectively withdraw from the service user. The effort of trying to induce or suppress their own emotional reactions, triggered by counter-transference, can contribute to compassion fatigue. Counter-transference as the name suggests can also be an attempt to 'counter' transference from a service user. So a service user may transfer past experiences onto the worker and the worker then projects an emotional response generated by this, and complicated by previous experiences, back onto the service user.

I had an experience of counter-transference when I was undertaking my doctoral research. In one of my focus groups with older adults, one man began to show irritated behaviour that reminded me of my father. In later years, my father, who had vascular dementia, would lose interest in a conversation or activity and exit the room. At times this was done in a tense and volatile way and my family and I would employ a range of techniques to manage this. In the focus group I was aware that I was becoming distracted by this man's behaviour and was drawn to attempting to placate him as I would with my father to prevent the volatile behaviour. Being distracted ran the risk of me losing the focus of the wider discussion, which was going well. I acknowledged to myself that I was reminded of my father's behaviour, but this man was not my father. Instead, I drew on my own personal experience to utilise strategies to keep him engaged where possible, while accepting that he might not participate and that he could choose to walk out. I was then able to prevent his behaviour become a distraction for me, while still being respectful and attentive to him.

The man may have been having a reaction to previous experiences about struggling to partake in groups or not feeling heard, complicated by a hearing difficulty. He may have, through his own transference, then begun to project these earlier responses into this situation and I, from a different experience, reacted and tried to counter them.

Parallel process is a mirroring of emotional response first identified in supervision in psychotherapy where the therapist projected the feelings and reactions associated with a service user onto the supervisor and the supervisor began responding to these. Schamess (2006) notes that supervisees and supervisors may unconsciously replicate problematic relational patterns that supervisee enacts with clients (p. 429). If emotional reactions toward and from the service user are re-enacted in supervision by the supervisee, and the supervisor joins in these, a parallel process occurs.

An example of this was a worker in an organisation I worked for who was noticing strong feelings of hopelessness and helplessness when working with a client who was experiencing depression. The worker would come back to the office and find themselves crying and overwhelmed by the situation, a form of mirroring of the service user's emotional state. In a clinical supervision session with me, the worker became tearful in our conversation and I in turn felt briefly saddened and somewhat hopeless. I noticed these feelings surfacing and recognised a possible parallel process. In observing and sharing my own response to what the supervisee was experiencing I said, "When you were describing feeling stuck with this client, I found myself noticing my own mood drop a little, is this what is happening for you when you are working with them?" I also said, "I wonder if this feelings of stuckness is what your client is experiencing, what do you think?" They were able to see this, and that realisation created an immediate shift. They also named their own fear about not knowing how to 'fix' the situation and therefore failing. We were able to talk this through and develop some strategies, including then using their own emotional awareness and mindfulness techniques to stay in compassionate engagement but not join in the emotional experience of the client. This included maintaining a gentle positive and hopeful mood and energy while acknowledging how hard the experience was for the client.

A key indication of counter-transference or parallel process is the intensity and type of emotion being experienced in response to the person or situation. If a supervisee appears unduly heightened, reactive, or is experiencing a similar emotional response to that of the client, the supervisor aims to make this conscious. This helps with the therapeutic function of supervision by giving the supervisee insight and control back over their emotional reactions, effectively lessening the impact of these. The following questions are very helpful to surface and make transference and counter-transference conscious:

- What feelings come up for you when you are working with this person?
- Are these feelings strong, different or unusual for you to experience?
- Do you think they are experiencing any of those feelings?
- If they were an animal, what sort of animal would they be?
- What sort of animal are you like around them?
- What do you like about the person?
- What are you finding challenging about them?
- Do they remind you of anyone? (This could be a client, someone currently in your life, someone in your past).
- What role do you think they are expecting you to take with them?
- Do you feel an urge to avoid them?
- Is there something you want them to do or say?

- What do you think is their key issue?
- How can this reflection help you in your work with them?

(adapted Rothschild, 1993)

I particularly like the fourth and fifth animal questions which may seem unusual to ask (and I always prefix them with "We're not saying they are an animal, just what animal they remind you of") as they provide very valuable and useful information. I have asked these questions many times and the supervisee and I have often ended up laughing about their answers as their responses have included honey badgers, chubby teddy bears, sleek antelopes with pointy horns, and whales! But on a serious note, these questions help surface any counter-transference and help the supervisee see the situation in an externalised way. I also add a third question "What kind of animal would you like to be around them?" as this starts to invite a different future picture of engagement.

Counter-transference and parallel process provide an opportunity to express and explore what is happening emotionally and supervision is an ideal place to do this without unpacking deep seated psychodynamic issues. The supervisor role is to support self-identification of transferential dynamics, help the supervisee develop non-reactivity to these through awareness and articulation, process the emotions occurring in the present moment, and move back into engagement if this has become affected. If they have a persistent strong counter-transference, they may need to further explore this in a counselling space. This also applies to the supervisor.

By being critically aware of transferential dynamics, we have the potential to tap into these as a rich source of information, not only about the person we are working with but also ourselves. This requires us to listen closely to our emotions, thoughts, feelings, and body responses to people. We need to check if what we are experiencing belongs fully to this situation or could in part belong to older experiences we have had. Parallel process and counter-transference provide powerful sources of emotional information and excellent opportunities for reflection and enhanced insight which can help reduce emotional impact of the work.

Transactional analysis

Previous emotional responses and coping strategies that people use, especially as children, may have been adaptive and worked at that time, but as people grow older, can become maladaptive and contribute to alienation and people withdrawing from interaction with them. Eric Berne's transactional analysis theory developed in the 1950s, explores three different ego states: child, adult, and parent, and suggests people might move in and out of these in interpersonal interactions or 'transactions'. Berne (1958) noted that people who came from a history of relational trauma as children often become caught in the ego positions of child and parent and unconsciously move others into these roles as well, instead of engaging with others from an 'adult' to 'adult' interaction. Again, driven from insecure attachment styles shaped by early unmet needs, people often experience unstable and unsatisfactory adult relationships because of continuing childhood patterns of attempting to get needs met rather than having constructive ways of navigating this in an adult way.

Alternatively, people might use authoritarian or overly directive ways of trying to get their needs met based on what adults did when they were children (shouting, threatening, withdrawing) so be in a 'critical parent' rather than adult state. Being in an adult state is an objective and more reasoned way of naming and exploring healthy ways to have needs recognised and met. This comes from the transactional position of "I'm ok, you're ok" rather than of "I'm not ok, you're ok" (positioning self as lesser) or a power over of "I'm ok, you're not ok", with the least helpful being "I'm not ok, you are not ok", which creates a defeated and defensive position from which to face the world.

The Drama Triangle (Karpman, 1972) and a counter model to this, The Empowerment Dynamic (Emerald & Zajonc, 2013) also explore transactional analysis. In the drama triangle workers take positions of victim (the primary role), rescuer (acting to 'save' the victim usually without being asked) and persecutor (attacking or keeping the person in victim) within relationships where conflict and difficulty exist. These positions are usually based on past transferred issues of shame and not having had their needs well met or understood. In the rescuer position, workers enact a need of being wanted, in victim they abdicate responsibility, and in persecutor they apply blame to manage the discomfort in relationship. Two people can move around the triangle, often unconsciously playing out these roles. Supervision is an ideal place to surface where a supervisee may be caught in the drama triangle, the clue being the word drama, so persistent interactions which are dramatic in description.

The Empowerment Dynamic moves a person from interacting from a victim state into one of 'creator', where they are future focused and looking to create solutions by taking ownership of their own life direction in the interaction. Instead of aligning with a person in a victim role in the drama triangle and 'rescuing' them, a person can choose a role of 'coach', where they support the person to find their own solutions and walk alongside them to do this. Finally, by moving from a persecutor role to being a 'challenger' instead, a person focuses on their own self-assertiveness, focusing on contributing to positive change, and pushing ahead for solutions.

Another influencing factor in adult transactions that may play out in dynamics such as the drama triangle, are early attachment styles. People who experienced an avoidant attachment with adults as child, may distance themselves or withdraw from others. This is based on their experience of being let down by adults who failed to meet their needs and may in fact have silenced these. The child learns to not rely on others and can find emotional intimacy difficult and uncomfortable as an adult, often preferring to withdraw as a form of self-protection. Children who experienced an anxious attachment style, learn that adults are unpredictable and the child experiences confusion, uncertainty, and anxiety in the context of relationships. In adult relationships, they may pursue certainty to ease the anxiety developed from the lack of predictability they experienced as a child. At its worst, the pursuer/withdrawer dynamic (identified in Emotion Focused Therapy) underpins intimate partner violence, where the two sets of insecure attachment styles with unmet needs collide and frequently explode.

This pursuer/withdrawer dynamics can be seen in workplaces, where one worker feels anxious in their own belonging and may pursue another colleague as a form of getting relief from these feelings. If this person happens to have an avoidant style, this can feel overwhelming and they will withdraw, or strongly push back resulting in conflict. Until the pursuer/withdrawer dynamic is surfaced, it will likely keep repeating itself.

I had a supervisee caught in a version of the drama triangle and a pursuer/withdrawer dynamic with a colleague. This relationship was a persistent topic in supervision (a clue that some sort of transactional relationship difficulty is occurring) with my supervisee expressing stress and even distress from the interactions. They alternated between feeling like a victim, then reacting to this and being persecutory, and finally at times rescuing the colleague in other work contexts. Their colleague also moved around the triangle with them. In supervision we identified and named the dynamics and set of transactions that were paying out between them which immediately brought illumination to the issue. This included coaching my supervisee to gently bring awareness of this to the colleague. We then explored ways for my supervisee to remain in coach, challenger, and creator role instead, namely creator, as victim was the primary role they were taking.

With some practice, and noticing when they re-entered the drama triangle, they both managed to remain out of it by recognising each other's strengths, combined successes and maintaining a focus on the future work they wished to achieve rather than becoming lost in the drama of the past difficulties. There was also a pursuer/withdrawer dynamic underpinning this working relationship stemming from their individual early attachment styles. Recognition of this helped further externalise the two sets of behaviour, providing for a commitment to recognise and not engage in their early learnt behaviour, instead staying with 'I'm ok, you're ok' in their communication.

The problem is the problem not the person

The strength-based practice principle of the 'problem is the problem not the person' provides an opportunity to defuse high emotion in relational interactions. Essentially a form of externalising, it can help a supervisee separate the problem from the person and to gain better clarity on the actual issue. If we meld a problem with a person, it becomes very easy to label the person in a certain way and this quickly can become 'othering' where we see the person as different and problematic. Labelling people as their behaviour also contributes to a sense of feeling stuck in a relationship where the problem can feel insurmountable. By inviting a supervisee to firstly name the behaviour they are experiencing from the other person and give this detail, we start to identify the problem away from the person and we can then explore how to best address it. This includes identifying with the supervisee how they respond to the problem and what is helpful and perhaps not so helpful about this.

I allow space and time for the supervisee to express their reaction, usually frustration, anger and disappointment, so these emotions are given space, voice, and can begin to disperse. I check for any older life scripts, ordering principles, counter-transference and parallel process that might be driving these responses which helps the supervisee take responsibility for their reaction. I then ask them to hypothesise why they think the person might be behaving in this way, which supports the development of compassion which will be explored in the next chapter. We examine what they have tried, what has worked, and what else might help. I always emphasise that we cannot change another person, but we can change how we respond to their behaviour, so the impact of it is reduced for us. For most people who work in human service work, being able to move out of strong negative reactions toward a person by clearly seeing the problem as the problem rather than the person themselves, sits more comfortably with their intention of fairness, acceptance, empathy, and compassion.

It can also be helpful to apply metaphors to support externalising of an issue, and to enable a supervisee develop insight and a different perspective on this. We can invite the supervisee to apply a metaphor to the situation, what does it look like, feel like, or remind them of? We can ask them to draw the issue in the form of a shape or object. We can also apply the concept of a metaphor in the exploration of feelings, so we learn more about the impact of it through the use of metaphoric description. Being able to visualise the situation in the form of something, gives us ways to then look at how the impact could be reduced and the future picture of how they would want it to be.

Another form of externalising, particularly when looking at relational issues, is to invite the supervisee to imagine what the other person might be feeling and or what they might say about what is happening. We can invite them to literally sit in a different chair in the supervision room and hypothesise from that seat what might be happening for the other person. We then invite them back into their seat, and hence themselves, and reflect on whether the exercise on stepping into the other person's perspective has changed anything for them or given them some insight on how to best manage it. Even the smallest reframe can shift perspective and create movement from a point of feeling stuck, stressed, distressed, and reactive.

Summary

The examination of relational dynamics contributes to the therapeutic function of supervision and can increase self-awareness and understanding which relieve stress. Self-awareness, self-knowledge and a commitment to personal and professional development are essential for best practice, and the examination of relationships richly informs this. As supervisors we must also examine the relational dynamics in our supervisory relationships and look for the places of learning in these. Engaging the therapeutic function of supervision brings us closer to people's energy, including pain and hope. This in turn may at times bring us closer to our own difficult experiences, both from the past and in the present. It is essential that we know ourselves before trying to know someone else, and that we remain open to the powerful wisdom that the experience of being in relationships with others brings us.

References

Atwood, G. E., & Stolorow, R. D. (1993). *Faces in a cloud: Intersubjectivity in Personality theory.* New Jersey: Jason Aronson, Inc.

Berne, E. (1958). Transactional analysis: A new and effective method of group therapy. *American Journal of Psychotherapy, 12*(4), 735–743.

Connolly, M., & Harms, L. (2009). *Social work. Contexts and practice.* 2nd Edition. Sydney: Oxford University Press.

Dewane, C. (2006). Use of self, a primer revisited. *Clinical Social Work Journal, 34*(4), 543–558.

Edwards, J., & Bess, J. (1998). Developing effectiveness in the therapeutic use of self. *Clinical Social Work Journal, 26*(1), 89–105.

Emerald, D., & Zajonc, D. (2013). 'TED'. Making the shift from drama to empowerment. https://cbodn.wildapricot.org/Resources/Documents/2013%20Conference/Power%20of%20TED%20Summary%20Two%20Sided%202013_Tso.pdf. Downloaded 8 September 2022.

Karpman, S. (1972). Fairy tales and script drama analysis. Downloaded from https://karpmandramatriangle.com/pdf/DramaTriangle.pdf.

Hawkins, P., & Shohet, R. (2012). *Ebook: Supervision in the helping professions.* Berkshire: McGraw-Hill Education.

Rothschild, B. (1993). Transference & countertransference: A common-sense perspective. Cited in Haines, S. 2021. Exploring body centred countertransference. https://bodycollege.net/exploring-body-centred-countertransference/.

Rotter, J. B. (1954). *Social learning and clinical psychology.* Englewood Cliffs, NJ: Prentice-Hall.

Schamess, G. (2006). Transference enactments in clinical supervision. *Clinical Social Work Journal, 34*(4), 407–425.

Sudbery, J. (2002). Key features of therapeutic social work: The use of relationship. *Journal of Social Work Practice, 16*(2), 149–162. Downloaded by [University of Auckland library] 6 March 2016.

Weld, N., & Appleton, C. (2008). *Walking in people's worlds: A practical and philosophical guide to social work.* Auckland: Dunmore Publishing.

Weld, N. (2017). *E ko te matakahi maire therapeutic social work. Stand children services.* Tū Māia: Wellington.

6 Connecting to compassion

Committing to a compassionate (and courageous) approach in human service work supports engagement, understanding, and ultimately greater connection both to others and ourselves. Compassion should underpin every level of human service work including organisational structures. Supervision provides an ideal place to explore and engender compassion especially when there are strong reactions and feelings to a person or family, particularly negative ones. If not examined, these often counter-transference responses can lead to a rigid positioning in relation to a person, stress, possible judgement, and an inability to move forward.

The supervisee may also be engaged in significant emotion labour to suppress these reactions and induce a response that is professionally acceptable. Supporting the application of compassion to social service work, reduces this emotional labour as identified by Miller and Sprang (2017) who suggest that generating 'radical compassion' can help counter this. Compassion can reduce the surface acting of producing an emotional state for another person and contribute to professional fulfilment and rewarding connection.

Supervisors can also help workers practice self-compassion which can in turn reduce stress and promote wellness. In this chapter an applied definition of compassion is provided and further analysis of each component of it is explored in greater detail, along with the concept of self-compassion and self-forgiveness.

Defining compassion

Most consistent in definitions of compassion is the emphasis on noticing, recognising, and responding to suffering with the motivation to reduce or alleviate it, and the tolerance of uncomfortable feelings in ourselves. Nickson, Carter, and Francis (2019) comment

DOI: 10.4324/9781003359036-7

that "compassion is a concept, feeling, action, philosophy, belief and motivation known to humans throughout history" (p. 175). They also note that there is minimal literature on compassion in supervision, and contest that a compassionate approach in supervision would support the worker to critically reflect on their work with clients and improve engagement and effectiveness (Nickson, Carter & Francis, 2019). Compassion can be defined as the intentional commitment of developing understanding, demonstrating acceptance, and providing connection with the overall intention to reduce, alleviate or transform suffering.

An applied definition of compassion helps identify the various steps and stages to enable it. Compassion begins with self-awareness of our own reactions, beliefs, and values. We may need to emotionally regulate and anchor ourselves to core motivations and beliefs that support our integrity. We then consciously engage to demonstrate acceptance and develop understanding. Our intention is to enable connection and contribute to the alleviation or transformation of suffering which is demonstrated through action.

Compassion differs from empathy which begins with feeling, perceiving or sensing another person's emotions. Empathy is the joining and connecting with the emotional experience of another and brings us into closer relationship with them. This is based primarily on our own emotional experiences which may draw us to some people but perhaps not to others. It may or may not lead to an action to alleviate suffering. Because it has a strong emotional sensing aspect to it, it can literally be felt, and this can happen rapidly, sometimes in an unconscious way. This means it can be subjective and people may end up caught in the emotional experience of another person through unconsciously joining their own experience to that of the person. If not well regulated, it can become fatiguing and overwhelming.

Compassion involves a cognitive process that is conscious and deliberate. It begins with empathetic observation, but brings thinking to this, including wondering and considering which help build understanding. It may not require drawing on our emotional experience or the joining with that of the other person, but holds an intention of connection. Compassion is restorative as it can provide a sense of achievement and reward for making a connection to another person and contributing to a reduction in their suffering.

Compassion is purposeful and responsive, as it involves reflection and consideration of what may be happening. It does not contain pity which can constitute sympathy (Nickson, Carter & Francis, 2019). Compassion assists workers to notice the emotions present in a situation without becoming overwhelmed by them or joining with them.

By understanding each step and stage of the applied definition of compassion, we can help others and ourselves continue to cultivate and develop it.

Self-awareness

The first step to compassion begins with our self-awareness, including noticing what strong reactions is this person's situation generating in me, what emotions and beliefs are surfacing? This requires mindful presence and attunement, which support self-awareness. Self-awareness contains the skills of foresight, intentionality, self-reactiveness, and self-reflectiveness, which in turn provide the ability to self-regulate and self-motivate (Lester, Vogelgesang, Hannah & Kimmey, 2010). If we are to attune to others we must also attune to our inner world. When we are faced with a person whose behaviour evokes a strong negative reaction in us, our first clue may be a desire to pull or move away from that person. We may find ourselves wanting to shut down the interaction. This could be due to uncomfortable feelings, such as distaste, disgust, or even abhorrence. Our natural inclination may be to remove ourselves or avoid the situation. In doing so, we position the person as 'other', so separate from us, and this may reinforce years of rejection and disconnection for them. 'Othering' is a very young developmental step, where we form beliefs of good and bad, however maturity tells us behaviour alone should not define a person.

With confronting behaviour, we need to pay attention to our prejudice, fear, the desire to pull away and 'other'. We need to look deeply into ourselves and analyse the cultural lens we are looking at the situation through including privilege and conscious and unconscious bias. Committing to compassion invites us to pause and firstly bring our attention to our reactions, not suppressing them but observing them. This creates the pause between reacting and responding and helps keep us in relationship with the person.

I was in San Francisco and had just finished a day of teaching with social workers. I walked out of the building with two of the friendly teaching academy staff who had supported me through the day, and we headed along the street. We walked past an older man who was wearing torn unwashed clothes and was begging on the footpath with his small black and white dog. I looked at him as we passed and felt a tug of sadness in myself, along with a small edge of fear as he had a hard look to him. I noticed my fear and how it made me want to increase my foot speed. I considered that many people probably reacted to him like this, and yet what was the evidence of him being dangerous?

That was my projection based on how he looked. My two colleagues did not even look at him, perhaps so used to seeing homeless people around the streets.

I felt uncomfortable in myself about how I reacted, and I wondered about his daily life in the world and how it would be to be so unseen or judged. I also felt worried for his small patient dog sitting beside him. I slowed down, stopped, and then put down my laptop bag and found a couple of dollars in my wallet. My companions also stopped and I asked if they could look after my bag as I wanted to give the guy some money for food for his dog and I then ran back to the man. I held out my two dollars and to him and said maybe he could buy something for his dog. He mumbled thanks and did not make any eye contact. I smiled at him, said goodbye, and headed back to the two staff I was with. One of them laughed and said, "You realise you just threw your money away, he won't spend it on the dog". I picked up my bag and said "Well, he might".

It is ok to notice the urge to distance ourselves but in noticing this, we need to ask ourselves why. Is there a fear I hold that I might somehow become like this person? Could my life change and I find myself living a life like theirs? Do they remind me of a time in my life that I am not proud of? Do they remind me of my privilege and that feels uncomfortable? What value judgements are filling my mind about this person? What right do I have to hold these? This process of meta cognition where we take time to think about our thinking, our feelings, and reactions, helps us claim these responses as ours, and in fact, nothing to do with the person.

Everything we are feeling in that moment is a cumulation of story and beliefs from our experience. None of those belong to this person in front of us, and instead our responses offer us a glimpse into the everyday reality of this person. They invite us to replace our thoughts of judgement with thoughts of wondering – "I wonder what their life is like each day, it seems hard, what daily struggles do they face?" "If my life had been different, I too could be in that position". Once we are aware of our thoughts and feelings, we can replace them with other ones that help us approach and engage with a person. Through self-awareness we become present, and this means we can lean into social awareness of others.

Emotional regulation

Compassion requires 'distress tolerance', the ability to tolerate difficult emotions in oneself when confronted with someone else's suffering without becoming overwhelmed by them (Gilbert, 2009). In compassion we recognise the suffering of a person, which may be initially triggered by an empathetic awareness, but we do not join in this. This is a key difference between compassion and empathy which as noted, if not regulated well can cause us emotional distress. While empathy may take us into the emotional experience of another person, compassion brings a degree of observation where we recognise their experience to being unique to them and we cannot ever fully know how this feels.

Our reactions of fear, distaste, revulsion, anger, sadness all help provide emotional knowledge about the person's daily world and through firstly recognising these reactions, we can then regulate these. By inviting thoughts of wondering about how a person's world might be, we look at the behaviour in a different way, one that is rational rather than reactive. This helps turn the emotional reaction down in ourselves. We can wonder how a person's early childhood experiences has contributed to their adult behaviour as underpinning abusive behaviour is often a lifetime of pain, trauma, and loss of belonging. This is not about condoning or excusing behaviour, but instead helping us regulate our emotional reaction which could spill out in judgement or a projection of our beliefs and values.

Instead this type of wondering helps transform an emotion such as anger or revulsion into a softer one such as sadness. I wonder how their life has brought them to this point, I imagine them as a child, and what happened to them. The perpetuation of pain and unmet needs from those around them has most likely contributed to the expression of pain through the behaviour I am observing. I wonder about the life opportunities that never came for them or were taken away. I consider the understandable patterns of unhelpful coping they now lean on; drugs, addiction, risk taking, hurting others before they hurt you. All of these thoughts help me regulate my response and lean in rather than lean away.

The fundamental question of "What has happened to you?" spoken internally and then externally at some stage, shifts us from reaction to response. Shifting from judgement to curiosity softens or mitigates emotions of distaste, horror, revulsion. We can wonder, how has this person come to behave like this? What is their story? We can lean into gratitude for our reality versus theirs, realise that this could have been any of our lives but for the circumstances we were born into. We can also apply grounding through bringing attention to our breath and senses and use the energy of the earth to hold us steady and help us stand and be with what is.

We can book time to have our emotional expression where we give voice to our strong emotions we have contained. We can request debrief time straight away with a colleague, we can use supervision to fully express what we felt, so this too is heard and honoured. In supervision, giving time for the emotional expression will better enable the supervisee to regulate and shift their reaction into a softened place. Once our emotional reactions are expressed and settled, we can reach our higher cognition to bring us back into connection and find learning. It is important as a supervisor that we give space to these strong feelings and do not judge them, instead allow them to be named and given release.

Anchor to core motivation

Engaging in self-awareness and then emotional regulation requires an intentional purpose and this tends to be informed by our motivation to undertake the work we do. This is likely informed by core beliefs such as a commitment to social justice and upholding the humanity and dignity of all. For me this is about believing that every person arrived with a sacredness of spirit; that they are a unique and special person, worthy of respect and dignity. This is upholding the unique spirit in each of us that was there when we took our first breath. It is about seeing someone for who they were born to be, not who they became through harm and hurt.

It is also committing to an ethical course of action that upholds the beliefs and values of my profession. This recognises that I represent not just myself but all other social workers and that through my actions I commit to upholding and living the principles that inform my profession such as social justice, equity, human rights, respect and dignity.

When working cross culturally we look for similarity rather than difference. Fairfield (2013) suggests cross cultural challenges are mostly due to tracking unfamiliar or unexpected signals from others. We need to allow space for the person's narrative where our role is to listen and observe where we can 'transcend what is unfamiliar and build more shared ground'. This requires a commitment to uphold our core motivations and beliefs with everyone we work with, to find a point of commonality, and be willing to experience and learn.

Ultimately in human service work we aspire to alleviate and transform suffering for all. This requires bringing compassion to all, not selecting who may or may not receive this. I find connecting to my core motivations helps anchor me and hold me steady in situations that are emotionally volatile and difficult. They form the backbone of my work that keep me strong, that help me lean in and also remain anchored to what may need to happen to increase safety and address danger and harm. In every interaction, we have the opportunity to provide a relationship that contains healing and offers hope.

Consciously engage to develop acceptance, understanding and connection

The next step of compassion is to consciously engage, it is here where our attention that has been attuned inward now turns outward to the person. We actively engage and include them through a demonstrated acceptance of the person. We recognise and celebrate diversity and divergence but uphold safety. We stand and commit to social justice through the action of taking time to see the person, and apply the concept of tēnā koe – a Māori greeting that extends a willingness to see another person for the sacred person they are. The use of externalising helps to ensure we see the person not as their problem but with a problem. We engage by conveying hope that every person is capable of growth of change, and the role of judgement does not sit with us.

The conscious practice of 'non-judgement' is to remain accepting of and tolerant towards another person even when their condition gives rise to difficult feelings in oneself, such as frustration, anger, fear, or disgust. Compassion means approaching those who are suffering with non-judgement and tolerance even if they are in some sense disagreeable to us (Gilbert, 2009). This also includes the skill of reframing our perspective. A judgement often levelled at children with difficult behaviour is labelling this as 'attention seeking'. A simple reframe of this that drops judgement is seeing the behaviour as 'attention needing'. This invites a wondering of what unmet need are they trying to show us and how we can support these.

Miller and Sprang call this developing a "model of mind" of the client, where we wonder about the cognitive skills the client may lack rather than judging their motivations which will give rise to judgement in us (Miller & Sprang, 2017). We can then work with the service user to help them acquire skills that will support problem solving. When bringing a non-judgemental attitude, we still need to discern, assess, make a determination of risk and take action in relations to dangerous behaviour in order to protect a person and those around them, but this is different from judging a person, something no one has the right to do.

When we consciously engage, we step forward and begin the simplest of connection by looking at someone in their eyes. If they do not make eye contact, if there is shame, or fear, or anger, then we will respect this, but still hold that intent. We can ask questions and show listening that says we are interested, that we want to understand. A way to do this is to identify a point of connection/commonality, such as, "My friend has a black and white dog, what's your dog's name?" We are now moving into connection through which to develop acceptance and demonstrate understanding.

I had an example of a supervisee who spent a whole day with a man who was mentally unwell, and with his agreement she took him to the emergency department. During the six hour wait for him to be seen, he was at times verbally abusive, rude, shouting out, and disruptive. In an effort to calm him, my supervisee would ask him simple questions about his life to help redirect his thinking. At one point she asked him what his favourite food was, and she shared that hers was pasta. When they finally left the hospital she drove him back to his temporary shelter and gave him a food parcel. She walked with him to the door and as he went inside, he turned and asked her to wait. He then went inside and rummaged through the food parcel, re-appearing at the door holding out a bag of dried pasta. "This is for you", he said, "You said you like pasta".

I was so struck by this story that I asked her permission to share it as it highlighted both compassion and courage. Despite hours of very challenging behaviour, she was able to keep engaging with him and through this connection he was then able to reciprocate. This was despite being very unwell, and having had a life of severe trauma, addiction, abuse, and rejection. Showing interest, sharing a little of ourselves back, helps builds connection. There is a Maori proverb (whakataukī) which considers the impact of shame and disconnection:

> Kia aata akiaki i ahau, he kai ka mate kei te hara o te kakii.
> Dwell not on my faults, for the desire for food dies at the throat of sin.
> There is a point at which continual censure causes such shame that one can no longer eat and can therefore no longer make a contribution to the people. After this there is only suicide and death.
>
> (Williams, 1908, in Mead & Grove, 2021, p. 208)

Compassion provides space for a person's trauma narrative to be spoken and for us to deeply and fully listen. We can show understanding that abuse, neglect, and violence teach cruelty and that people end up feeling so alone that pain and hurt becomes their only point of control and power. Through conscious engagement and the demonstration of acceptance and understanding, we can develop a compassionate pathway to support safety.

It was also important for the supervisee to be able to openly discuss and share some of her reactions and thoughts during this situation to be able to put them out in the supervisory safe space. We do not want supervisees to surface act, suppress, or highly edit their responses to us as supervisors as this only induces more emotional labour for them. I encourage supervisees to freely name what they were feeling, and this can include swearing and being upset. The supervision session becomes the container for this, rather than the supervisee having to continue to work hard to suppress. Supervision is a professional relationship and supervisees will be aware of behaving in professionally acceptable ways, therefore trust is required in order for supervisees to be able to honestly share at this level. While, racist or other discriminatory outbursts would remain offensive, personal emotions such as anger and frustration are valid and provide an opportunity for further exploration and understanding.

Seppala, Rossomando, and Doty (2013) observes that people who feel more connected to others have lower rates of anxiety and depression. They are also likely to have higher self-esteem, are more empathic to others, more trusting and cooperative, and, consequently, others are more trusting and cooperating with them. Social connectedness therefore generates a positive feedback loop of social, emotional, and physical wellbeing (Seppala, Rossomando & Doty, 2013). Compassion invites us to look for places where a person's story may resonate with us and notice how and why. We can use this information to convey understanding and explore how they have survived and reinforce these strengths to help them continue forward.

I had a supervisee who wanted to explore in supervision how they felt 'irritated' by service users who did not appear to want to help themselves. They were feeling judgemental of a particular service user and did not like this response in themselves. They wanted to explore what generated this and how to reduce the irritation.

I invited them to tell me what had happened, and they shared that during the current COVID 19 lockdown the service user had demanded the supervisee do their shopping for them or at least collect and drop off a food parcel. My supervisee went through a few possible solutions and ideas the person could try to do this for themselves but felt these were all blocked. In the end the situation was left with the service user to try other supports and if none of these worked to get back to my supervisee. My supervisee expressed their view that people should try and solve their own problems and not wait for someone else to do this. My supervisee also identified their internal irritation was not helped by a recent stressful personal life event.

After I had invited the telling of what had happened and we had explored the irritation in more detail by my asking them what it felt like, and what emotions were a part of it, I invited them to develop a compassionate lens to view the situation through. We began this by firstly separating the client from their behaviour and we discussed the idea of the internal and external locus of control, concepts they had not heard of. I then asked them to consider what might have happened in the life of a person who has a high external locus of control, and they reflected on possible early trauma, attachment difficulties, anxiety, and not being assisted to develop problem solving skills as a child.

This began a different way of starting to see this person and I then asked them to consider if they thought there was worry, stress or distress sitting behind the demanding tone to the request that was made. They thought for a moment and reflected that yes, definitely there was some sort of stress and anxiety. My supervisee wondered if the person was being triggered into a fight flight freeze response and this was driving their demanding behaviour.

I then asked them to consider if they had given time to acknowledge the feelings that might be at play for the service user, so these were fully heard before moving to problem solving began. My supervisee paused and said that no, perhaps they had not given enough time to check in emotionally with the person but rushed to problem solving. We talked through how they could have done this differently, and also what compassionate statement they could say to themselves on hearing the more demanding tone of voice that triggered irritation in them. My supervisee was able to do this, and I asked if saying it helped with the irritation, and they identified it greatly softened this. We then discussed some other ways to support capacity building for the service user before they were discharged from the programme.

I then checked back in regarding how they were managing their own personal life event, and they shared how they had said to their manager that they felt they had very little to give prior to the lockdown. This made me wonder about some degree of compassion/empathy fatigue and I named this, and we talked about personal depletion of energy and how they might be able to replenish or top this up drawing on what had previously helped. I commented that given their life event, there was a great invitation to invite self-compassion for themselves and acknowledged how well they had managed the interaction with the person despite feeling depleted and irritated. I again acknowledged and affirmed their coping skills, and in our evaluation of the session, the supervisee named feeling better about the situation, lighter in themselves, and had some new techniques to apply to practice.

Self-compassion and self-forgiveness

While compassion provides a key way to address emotional labour, keeps us in relationship with people, and ultimately supports the alleviation of pain and suffering, workers also need to direct compassion toward themselves. Self-compassion has been found to reduce stress, trauma impacts and compassion fatigue (Miller, Lee, Chunling, Grise-Owens & Bode, 2019, p. 3), along with increasing life satisfaction and overall wellbeing. Showing kindness and understanding toward oneself is more likely to result in engaging in rejuvenating and restorative activities and practices that evidence caring and a commitment to one's wellbeing. This would include reflective supervision and accessing other professional supports as required.

Self-compassion is a helpful strategy to apply when a worker makes a mistake or regrets how they have responded. This can lead to significant stress and distress which left unexplored and unintegrated can haunt workers through rumination, regret, and unresolve. Due to the complexities and challenges of working with a wide range of people in often resource comprised environments, mistakes in practice do happen. It can be difficult and devastating to live with a decision taken or an action resulting in a serious or potentially serious outcome. Becoming mentally and emotionally 'stuck' about a mistake can also lead to self-doubt, which in turn can erode confidence and lead to more errors.

One way of managing the emotional impact of a practice mistake is for us to 'self-forgive' ourselves. Although self-forgiveness is an individual task, supervision can play a key role in supporting this through the therapeutic function. This includes exploring the incident and the emotions and thoughts connected to it, examining the intent and motivation for the action taken, and providing feedback about it.

Enright (1996) comments that self-forgiveness is not required for matters that may provoke uneasiness, but rather for those events that provoke guilt, remorse and shame, and that it is not an "opiate for the pain, rather self-forgiveness leads us into the pain before it leads us out" (Enright, 1996, p. 118). Dillon (2001, p. 58) also comments that if a person is not bothered by it or is bothered but gets over the event, the need to forgive oneself is not required. A supervisee once said to me, "Shame took over and I put myself in a dark corner". It is those experiences that are likely to require self-forgiveness and a supervisor can help with this. Being present with an experience also requires us to resist criticising, changing or judging it. This includes not pushing away feelings and instead being aware and curious of them.

Self-reproach is another indicator for the need for self-forgiveness. Self-reproach suggests a process of self-examination, whereby a person recognises that they have let themselves down, according to their standards, morals, and values, and this has affected their self-respect. Dillon (2001, p. 75) comments that overcoming something is not about eradicating it but "we can overcome things by not letting them cripple or control us, by lessening or constraining their power over us". Therefore, a supervisor will be looking for indicators of mistakes that continue to dominate a worker's thinking in ways that are causing doubt, guilt, and shame and are impacting a worker's ability to practice confidently. Dillon also suggests that engaging in self-forgiveness is like being at a crossroad:

> There is reason to continue to view oneself as the kind of person who could do such things and there is reason to view oneself as a better person … to forgive oneself is to take the second road, to see oneself as a better person.
>
> (Dillon, 2001, p. 79)

This requires an acceptance of our fallibility at times while we still strive to live up to our values and retain confidence in our moral foundation and integrity. Munro (1996) comments that social workers need to have realistic and achievable standards of good practice, and that "making mistakes can be a sign of good practice, as a recognition of one's fallibility is part of a general willingness to be self-critical and to change one's mind" (pp. 2, 12). We each need to see ourselves as an inherently good person who made a poor or ill-informed decision, something that everyone does now and then. Learning from this is the most important task.

Self-compassion can also speak back to the inner critic or judge, a voice developed in childhood to remember 'what not to do' and to increase inclusion and belonging. While self-protective in childhood and stemming from a primal survival instinct to belong, this voice can be one of blame and intense shame when we are adults. The inner critic may be particularly strong in adults who as children experienced emotional and physical neglect, where they had to build an active critic to keep them safe as they did not get helpful cues about this. Adults who were highly criticised as children and developed self-blame for a lack of love or being seen, will likely have a louder inner critic as adults.

The inner critic when left unchecked can cause a person to go to war internally with themselves. It needs to be understood with compassion and curiosity as to what it is still trying to protect, and replaced with positive messages of self-truth such as "I tried, I'm a good person", "people make mistakes". We can acknowledge the critic for trying to protect us, but turn the volume right down, preferably off, on a voice that berates and causes us additional emotional suffering. Instead we can replace this voice with one of acceptance, tolerance, warmth and kindness.

We can encourage a supervisee to talk to themselves as they would talk to someone that they cared about. Encouraging gentle noticing and reflection on thoughts, emotions, and reactions through the Acceptance Commitment Therapy approach helps to give them voice but not let in the inner critic with its judging tone. Showing compassion to ourselves through self-directed kindness is much more likely to help than this critical voice from a past stage of our lives.

I had a supervisee share that they were feeling significant guilt over a person that they had just started to work with who seriously injured their child. The agency had known the family for some time and another worker leaving had resulted in the parent being transferred to my supervisee. There were no indicators of previous harm. My supervisee had rung the parent on a Thursday and began the engagement process with them. They said they would check back the following week, and for the parent to call them if they needed anything before then. There were no indicators of what was to come, with the parent saying they were doing fine. The serious assault happened in the weekend before my supervisee was scheduled to reconnect with them on Monday. Since then, my supervisee had not been sleeping well, and was noticing increasing anxiety and hypervigilance.

I explored the guilt with my supervisee, gently undoing the various layers of thinking, and helping them to re-check what they had done. They regretted not calling again on the Friday although this had not been indicated. We discussed how this may have helped but how it may not have as well, due to the high likelihood of the assault being the result of sudden rage. I asked my supervisee that if the assault had not happened, whether they would be doubting anything they had done up to that point. They said no, and this reflection started to reassure them.

We then discussed the importance of the agency taking time to reflect and critically assess everything they had done, to identify any points of learning, to hopefully help prevent something like this ever happening again. I asked my supervisee if there was anything they wanted to help put in place to support the learning going forward. They had a couple of ideas and I reinforced that those would help honour the child and that was the best that we could do. I then gently but firmly invited her to put the guilt down, reiterating the good practice I could hear. My supervisee said they would be able to do this now. When we cannot change what has happened, the best we can do is identify any learning that will help us change a possible future outcome.

While helping supervises to show self-compassion, we also need to practice this as supervisors. In our supervisory practice we may inadvertently say the wrong thing, or misjudge a response. I can think of a number of occasions where I have exited a supervision session mentally kicking myself for a well-intended but misguided comment. Actively practicing self-compassion requires regular messages to ourselves, such as "we all get things wrong", "I didn't intend that to happen", "I'm a good person, it was a mistake that I will learn from". We notice that we have high expectations of ourselves and we do not want to let people down. It is acknowledging that we are human and may not always get something right. This includes addressing the 'inner critic' and also catching self-judgement and examining this without landing in shame or self-blame, instead reframing it from a place of self-kindness. This accepts fallibility, honours the good intent that was there, and through the use of critical reflection, taking the learning from it, then letting it go.

Sometimes a supervisee may become stuck on an issue that triggers old messages from childhood. It is appropriate to identify these issues or events in supervision and then suggest they may want to examine these with a social worker, counsellor, therapist, or psychotherapist. Taking these steps shows a commitment to our own personal growth and development and encourages self-actualising. Practicing self-compassion can help us to relax and accept ourselves more which allows us to be more open and available to others. Ultimately self-compassion supports personal wellness through a reduction in emotional labour, stress, and distress.

Summary

Compassion begins with self-awareness and helps anchor us to our motivation for being in our professions and roles. Compassion invites us to wonder about the daily world of a person and commits to understanding and connection. We invite and listen for the adult's trauma story that may never have been told or heard, and understand the eroding of empathy, and the development of cruelty and violence. Compassion invites us to look for the person before the hurt and the damage occurred, to see the sacred spirit they came into this life with. Through self-awareness we notice our responses, self-regulate, consciously make eye contact, are calm steady, use a warm tone of voice, and lean in. We step forward to partner for increased safety and well-being by offering even the smallest choice. We convey hope and belief that people are capable of change and help people identify how this will look to strengthen safety.

Compassion helps us remain steadfast in our responsibilities especially for those who are the most vulnerable and to not waver from this. For supervisees and ourselves we can practice self-compassion and forgiveness when we get something wrong or make a mistake. Supervision can offer a safe space for the mistakes to be explored, help the learning to be named, for the exhale to come, and the situation to be gently put down, not forgotten, but made sense of, and insights gained from it.

In practicing self-compassion we notice harsh or self-criticising comments, reduce negative self-bias, identify the inner critic, replace with kind gentler reframes (self-kindness). This supports emotional regulation promoting calm and contentment, and increases our capacity to self-soothe when stressed. We can normalise mistakes as part of the human condition and key to learning, and demonstrate loving kindness and care to ourselves. If we can do this for ourselves, we will have greater capacity to act compassionately in work and wider worlds.

References

Dillon, R. S. (2001). Self-forgiveness and self-respect. *Ethics, 112*(1), 53–83.
Enright, R. (1996). Counselling within the forgiveness triad: On forgiving, receiving forgiveness, and self-forgiveness. *Counselling and Values, 40*, 107–126.
Fairfield, M. (2013). The Relational movement. British Gestalt Journal. Vol. 22. No. 1. pp 22–35.

Gilbert, P. (2009). Introducing compassion-focused therapy. *Advances in Psychiatric Treatment, 15*(3), 199–208. DOI: 10.1192/apt.bp.107.005264.

Lester, P. B., Vogelgesang, G. R., Hannah, S. T., & Kimmey, T. (2010). Developing courage in followers: Theoretical and applied perspectives. In C. L. S. Pury, & S. J. Lopez (Eds.), *The psychology of courage: Modern research on an ancient virtue* (pp. 187–207). Washington, DC: American Psychological Association.

Mead H, M., & Grove. N. (2021). *Nga Peepeha a ngaa Tiipuna. The sayings of the ancestors*. Wellington: Victoria University Press.

Miller, B., & Sprang, G. (2017). A components-based practice and supervision model for reducing compassion fatigue by affecting clinician experience. *Traumatology, 23*(2), 153–164. DOI: 10.1037/trm0000058.

Miller, J., Lee, J., Chunling, N., Grise-Owens, E., & Bode, M. (2019). Self-compassion as a predictor of self-care: A study of social work clinicians. *Clinical Social Work Journal, 47*(4), 1–15.

Munro, E. (1996). Avoidable and unavoidable mistakes in child protection work. *The British Journal of Social Work, 26*(6), 793–808.

Nickson, A. M., Carter, M.-A., & Francis, A. P. (2020). *Supervision and professional development in social work practice*. New Delhi Sage Publications Pvt. Limited.

Seppala, E., Rossomando, T., & Doty, J. R. (2013). Social connection and compassion: Important predictors of health and well-being. *Social Research: An International Quarterly, 80*(2), 411–430.

Williams, H. W. (1908). *He Whakataukī, he Titotito, he Pēpeha*. Gisborne: Te Rau Kahikatea.

7 Supporting courage, grit, and resilience

In human service work, the ideal partner to compassion is courage, which enables the facing of adversity. This is followed by the ability to endure adversity through grit, and adapt to it through resilience. Adverse situations cause a response of fear, vulnerability, doubt, and uncertainty, mainly regarding how a person will cope or manage. The therapeutic function of supervision applies the concepts of courage, grit, and resilience in order to support workers to manage adversity and strengthen themselves both professionally and personally. This in terms helps reduce the impact of future events by supervisees having greater internal resources to call on.

Each time we face, endure, and adapt to challenge, we become stronger and more equipped to tolerate and manage future difficulties. As supervisors, we can affirm when a supervisee has acted with courage, grit, and resilience through the exploration of how they responded or are responding. This is especially important when they are facing personal challenges as well as the complexities of work demands, where the supervisor effectively becomes part of the worker's support team. Maidment and Beddoe (2012) comment that "encouraging creativity within the supervision process is yet another strategy for building resilience and coping skills among a stretched and often stressed social service workforce" (p. 166). Supporting courage, grit and resilience help equip supervisees to better meet the demands of the work.

Courage, grit, and resilience also assist with work that carries exposure to traumatic experiences of clients, and can in itself be traumatic. There are times when workers may have to enter into situations that understandably generate fear and doubt. Human beings are not predictable, and the trajectory of trauma and disadvantage can contribute to behaviour that can be both confronting and frightening. Along with the emotional processing and development of a coherent

DOI: 10.4324/9781003359036-8

narrative, courage, grit, and resilience can help workers to remain engaged in this type of work. The application of courage, grit and resilience reduces the potential for Secondary Traumatic Stress and strengthens their ability to work safely with situations which generate fear and uncertainty.

Defining courage

I studied the concept of courage in my doctoral research and one of my research participants commented that social work and human service work frequently requires walking into the unknown. This includes situations that we can never be fully prepared for, and ones that are may be life changing. Human service work shows us the very best and the very worst of humanity, and offers us profound opportunities of experience and learning. To take up these opportunities often requires courage.

Another of my research participants said, "When you are showing courage you are on a journey you haven't accomplished yet, showing courage is taking part in that journey" (Jill). Like compassion, a commitment to face our work with courage provides an approach that underpins our practice. Joan Halifax, a Buddhist teacher applies the concept of having a 'soft front' and a 'strong back' in her palliative care work (Halifax, 2008). This is the ability to be strong and flexible, yet open and engaging in relationship. Compassion can be seen as having the soft front and open heart, while courage provides a strong back. Courage helps us face adversity, enabling us to step into adverse situations and see them through.

Courage does not have a universal definition, despite being a concept that has been around for hundreds of years. Often reserved for situations of heroic action, courage can be found in everyday situations, as one of my research participants said, "Facing everyday adversity requires quiet courage". We can see this in coping with life changing diagnoses or staying beside someone who is dying. Through my research I developed the following definition of courage:

> Courage is a way of responding to situations that generate fear, vulnerability, doubt and uncertainty. It involves a conscious and intentional undertaking of perceived meaningful and important action. The decision to undertake this action is motivated by values, beliefs, morals, duty, and responsibility. Courage is characterised through a number of traits, attributes and behaviours,

such as logical thinking, calmness, determination, acceptance, endurance and perseverance.

(Weld, 2019)

The first stage of courage is the recognition that we are facing an adverse situation. These situations generate fear, doubt, vulnerability, and uncertainty. They are the types of situations that leave us unsure about what to do, and our initial reaction may cause us to want to fight, or avoid through flight. Or we may freeze. It is likely we may never have faced something like this before. Adversity involves a threat to physical and psychological safety and our instinct may be to self-protect. Situations that do not contain fear or vulnerability for us either physically or psychologically do not require courage.

Once we recognise adversity, courage requires a conscious process to stay and face what is happening. Often courage is seen as an unconscious decision, say a person who ran into the fire to rescue the child without stopping to think, but there is always some thinking occurring. A conscious decision is always made to turn and face what is occurring rather than walk away or avoid it. In human service work we make the decision to walk into the unknown every day, that is courage. At some point we decide to do this despite the fear, doubt, vulnerability, or uncertainty we might be experiencing.

As with compassion, when we respond with courage, we have to anchor to motivations that counter our natural responses to not want to face what is happening. Motivations come from a variety of places, including our socialisation, beliefs, and values that are ingrained in us from childhood, and as professionals we develop ethics, roles, duty, responsibilities, and further values that uphold the commitment to service we have undertaken. It is very important to identify and understand values and beliefs and to check they serve both us and those we work with. Reflective supervision is key place to undertake this level of critical thinking.

The conditions of adversity that require courage are highly emotional. Fear, vulnerability, doubt, uncertainty are all emotions that can easily take over. Courage is shown when people take action in spite of these emotions. This is done through emotional regulation involving self-talk including connecting to core motivations that help us move forward. It is not about being without fear but being with the fear yet taking action. A number of my research participants shared having a sense of equanimity, where they acted calmly and logically when facing adversity, remaining composed in order to do what needed to be

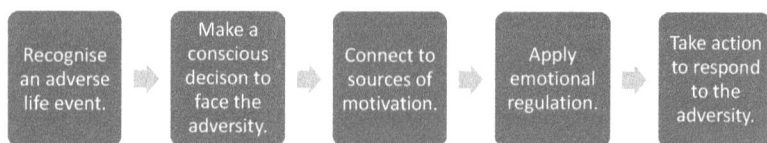

Figure 7.1 Process model of courage.

done. Finally the process of courage takes us into action. The stages of courage (which are very similar to the steps found in compassion) can be summarised in the process model (Figure 7.1):

Application to supervision

I had a supervisee who worked with children with significant relational trauma histories and very challenging behaviour. This included a recent number of highly distressing self-harm incidents. My supervisee was the on-call leader for these situations and identified in supervision that they were now having a noticeable physical startle reflex and feeling fearful when receiving an after hour call. On exploring these feelings and reactions further, they identified heaviness in their legs when thinking about walking into the facility and wanted to avoid doing so. My supervisee said they do not want to take the calls because they felt dread and fear.

What they were describing fit within an Acute Stress Disorder, and possibly Secondary Traumatic Stress, so in applying the reflective learning cycle, we took time exploring their emotional responses and giving voice to these to help develop a coherent narrative around what had happened, As we moved into the experimentation stage of the cycle, I asked them to think of an adverse situation in their life that they felt they had responded well to and that they did not mind sharing with me. They told me about some years ago having to bear witness to a sudden and traumatic loss of a loved one and support others around this. I used the process model of courage to explore and explain how they approached this previous adverse situation, unpacking and working through each of the steps within it.

By applying the process model of courage, we confirmed the adversity of the historical situation, we talked through how they made a conscious decision to go and offer support despite their fear and own distress, and we explored the motivating factors they called on to do this. We examined how they had mastered their emotions and what behaviours others might have displayed in the situation. This reflection confirmed that they had acted courageously.

We then used this information and the process model to explore how they could respond to future difficulties in their on-call role. We discussed the motivating sources they could draw on and ways to utilise them from their past experience to master their emotions. We talked about how they would behave in taking action, including ways to continue to demonstrate emotional mastery. In applying the process model we reinforced their capacity to act courageously, and we developed a plan to enact this to face future adversity. The supervisee identified this as very helpful and said their distress and fear had lifted through talking it all out and having their existing competencies affirmed and an approach and plan to work from.

Here are some reflective questions I use in supervision to support courage in practice. You can see each step of the process of courage in them.

Questions to connect courage

1 Is there an experience you can think of where you felt you coped with something frightening or uncertain?
2 In this experience, did you find yourself experiencing uncertainty, vulnerability or fear? Can you describe what your top three worries were?
3 It sounds like you made a conscious decision to act despite these feelings. Can you tell me what has motivated that for you?
4 When you talk about the motivating factors for deciding to act, how do these connect to your personal beliefs and values?
5 Tell me what you then did?
6 If someone else had been watching you, what attributes or behaviours would they have seen you enacting?

Woodard (2010) comments that choosing to live courageously can result in a "sense of wholeness, faith in living, a sense of identity, creativity, love, opening the opportunity for actualisation of one's true self" (p. 115) and to "live life less afraid" (p. 119). He notes that:

Self-actualised people are unafraid of the unknown, display calmness even in turbulent times, lack guilt, shame, and severe anxiety, and generally accept themselves for what they are. Self-actualised people are not defensive and dislike hypocrisy, game players, and any other attempts to impress others. They demonstrate a simple and natural spontaneity and 'play down' their unconventionality so as not to hurt others. They are spontaneous in their own style, and develop their own style by virtue of their self-knowledge.

(Woodard, 2010, pp. 117–118)

Courage is one of the greatest capacities available to us. Sometimes our humility stops us from recognising courage and compassion in our work, but it is important that we surface and articulate these concepts as by doing so will reinforce these skills for future use. The supervisory relationship should also contain the quality of courage, where experiencing vulnerability to critically assess oneself is celebrated and encouraged. This extends supervision from being a safe space to also a brave space. This should be for both supervisee and supervisor, as the presence of courage and compassion provide for mutual honesty, curiosity, learning, and connection.

Grit

When facing challenge or difficulty that is longer term in nature, we can support supervisees to act with grit. Along with courage, grit, hardiness, and fortitude all describe the traits needed for enduring difficulty and increase our tolerance and capacity to manage adversity. Grit is a way of coping and keeping on going in a difficult situation, portrayed through attitudes "commitment, control and challenge" (Maddi, 2004, p. 295). Seeing a difficulty as a challenge evidences an attitude of control whereby the difficulty is seen as an opportunity to develop, learn and see something through. In a difficult time, the attitude of control suggests a higher internal locus of control, where people identify what is in their control rather than becoming help-less and overwhelmed. Finally, the attitude of commitment is one of engaging with the difficulty and not avoiding it, instead seeing it through as a part of personal development.

Always returning to the familiar or avoiding discomfort or fear does not lead to self-development, only a confirmation of what is already known. The transformative nature of experience and the inte-gration of learning from this into knowledge is denied, and a return to the known is the only journey taken. It is not in the known that people grow; it is in the unknown. Learning is therefore expansive; it opens a person to both external and internal new information that expands self-knowledge and wider knowledge (Weld, 2019). By applying the therapeutic function in supervision, we are not only restoring but also strengthening for the future, and strength will more likely come when people embrace difficulty rather than avoid it.

Grit is evidenced through mental toughness, a concept most often applied in physical sports linked to the endurance. Mental toughness relies on management of thoughts and deliberate attention to thinking in ways that help a person push on and through. Negative thoughts easily help a person lose momentum and conviction in endurance events, and when the physical body is tiring it is the mental strength that will carry a person through to the finish line. This might involve distraction, so thinking about things that take the mind off the pain being experienced. It is about stopping thoughts such as "This is too hard, I'm too tired, I can't do this" and instead replacing them with ones such as "Look how well I'm doing, not far to go now, hey only a few kilometres left". It is largely about using our minds to focus on ways that will help not hinder, and to use mental discipline to do this. We remind ourselves of other tough situations we got through, we use self-encouragement and pay attention to what is happening around us in the present moment.

In supervision we can remind people of their ability to endure by exploring other situations where they saw a difficult situation through. We ask them how they did this, what got them through, and how did it feel to come out the other side. By reminding people of the qualities, capacities, and strengths they have accessed before, we re-connect them to these, as part of their equipment for the long road ahead. We can also explore in supervision what other 'equipment' they might need and how they can access this. This includes what helps them tolerate difficulty, and uncertainty, and the mental reserves they access to help with this. We also need to help a supervisee connect to the reason why they are seeing this adversity through, the motivation, what they hope to gain, what opportunities it might bring, and how it will contribute to their personal and professional growth. Just like with compassion and courage, we must act from motivations that matter to us which help us keep focused on seeing something through.

I had a supervisee who was working in a new organisation, where roles were unclear and anxiety not well named, all of which were persistently exhausting and difficult. However rather than leave, my supervisee was determined to see the role out for at least a year, citing the learning that could come from it, and their belief in the intention of the work. It helped for them to position the role as finite, so they did not feel despair, but we also explored what they were learning and noticing in terms of their own challenges and opportunities.

While they could have bailed out a lot earlier, they stuck with it, showing endurance built from seeing other difficult situations through, and embracing the often hard personal learning that presented through the position they were in. I kept a focus in our sessions of restoring and strengthening, in particular we talked often about them being their best self, and always responding with quiet dignity to the chaos and often poor behaviour from others. We cannot change other people, but we can still identify points of influence in situations, change our attitude and our approach, and cross the finish line at the end with our heads held high.

Resilience

The final stage of managing adversity is through the adaptive process of resilience. Rather than a set of fixed traits, resilience is best viewed as a "stable pattern of healthy adjustment" (Bonanno, 2012, p. 753) following adversity. Resilience is evidenced through positive adaptive coping strategies such as identifying what is within one's control, self-compassion, determination, tolerance, focusing on being present, and being able to notice what is positive or ok about a situation. It is the ability to recover from adversity with increased adaptive coping strategies that can be potentially applied to future challenges and difficulties. Adamson (2012) notes that resilience contains a 'matrix' of internal and external factors that "build the ability to withstand pressure and adapt over time" (p. 189).

We have a remarkable capacity for adaptation to life altering circumstances that occur outside of our control. Natural disasters and events such as the global pandemic, highlight how human beings can incorporate new ways of being and living to best respond to change and to help survive. People do better with adaptation when they understand what is occurring and what needs to happen in response to it. If we can keep and connect to some known, certain aspects of our lives, we are more able to make the transition of change that is required.

As with courage and grit, we can help people access resilience and continue to develop this, by the reminder and connection to existing strengths. In supervision we can ask a worker about a time that posed difficulty and challenge, and what helped them internally and externally manage this. We can help the supervisee mine these experiences for the resilient traits they showed in adapting to them. These might be humour, positivity, creativity, regulation of emotion, self-awareness, and solution finding so incorporating a future focus, calmness, determination, and optimism. We do not often put into words the resilience we have built up through life, and doing this with another person such as a supervisor, helps these to become articulated and tangible. The power of hearing yourself and then someone else name your strengths and positive coping strategies cannot be underestimated.

However, we should not rush to a conversation about resilience without having given adequate time and enabled a safe space for the strong emotions connected to adversity and life changing situations to be discussed. With any change there is always a degree of loss; loss of the known, loss of security, loss of stability, and of what is familiar. Even in times of positive and exciting change such as new job or a move to a different city or country, there will be losses to be grieved. If we rush someone past their loss and do not give adequate time for the expression of this, they may not make the transition quite so well. We can enquire about what they are looking forward to, and any worries or losses that they are identifying. It is after the expression of these that we can gently tap into previous ways they have managed and what helped.

A criticism levelled at resilience theory is when it is applied to inadvertently label people, for example, "They're resilient, they'll be fine" or "But you're so resilient, you'll manage it". If a person is not feeling resilient or struggling with this particular adverse experience, inadvertently labelling them in this way will deny their actual feelings of worry, struggling to cope, exhaustion and sadness. It may force people to put on a 'brave face' when they just want to fall apart for a little while. If they do fall apart when labelled 'resilient' this may cause a sense of failure that they did not manage as others assumed they would.

Labelling people as resilient may also inadvertently reduce resources made available to them instead seeing them as coping when they may not be. They may be left having to endure more than they can bear. Resilience is a combination of internal and external resources people have access to, not who they are, and sometimes in challenging and overwhelming situations they may not be able to access these (Bonanno 2012). Everyone needs time to grieve loss and change and to not have to be strong and coping all of the time.

I had a supervisee who was feeling extremely challenged by the behaviour of a new staff member. The situation was certainly not easy, and the behaviour was very disruptive and destabilising for those around this new team member. My supervisee was very upset about the situation and was naming distress, powerlessness, and anger in response to it. I gave lots of time for the expression of these emotions as they were valid and needed space to be heard. We also worked to clarify their position around the behaviour and to link this to clear service goals and principles, so it became less about personality and more about a lack of fit with the service. I would then gently steer the conversation to how they had managed previous difficulties in the team like this, and the strategies they used. We discussed times in their life when they had faced significant adversity which helped both bring perspective to this situation and remind them of previous positive adaptive ways they had already developed. This helped shift them to being able to keep facing into and enduring what was happening while adapting and managing it through having existing strength and resilience affirmed. Adamson (2012) notes that a supportive supervisory relationship itself can be a buffer against stress in challenging work environments (p. 192).

Summary

Supporting courage, grit, and resilience in supervision contributes to managing adversity in the present moment and building resource for facing this in the future. When facing adversity, a supervisee may feel out of their depth, with fear, doubt, vulnerability, and uncertainty, flooding in. Time to name and make sense of these feelings begins to clear these aspects and helps a way forward to be found. If the situation has passed, we can explore how they applied courage and grit, and through this, build a picture of their resilience with them. Doing this in supervision helps a person strengthen their skills, knowledge, and confidence for future adversity, by intentionally filling their resource pool of strengths and capacities. It is in the uncomfortable and challenging places that we grow and develop, learning more about ourselves and others. Facing, enduring and adapting to adversity provides invaluable learning and helps us recognise we are often stronger than we realise. Articulating and affirming this in supervision is another way of providing the therapeutic function.

References

Adamson, C. (2012). Supervision is not politically innocent. *Australian Social Work*, 65(2), 185–196. DOI: 10.1080/0312407X.2011.618544.
Bonanno, G. (2012). Uses and abuses of the resilience construct: Loss, trauma, and health related adversities. *Social Science and Medicine*, 74(5), 753–756.

Halifax, J. (2008). *Being with dying: Cultivating compassion and fearlessness in the presence of death.* Boston: Shambhala Publications.

Maddi, S. R. (2004). Hardiness: An operationalization of existential courage. *Journal of Humanistic Psychology, 44*(3), 279–298. DOI: 10.1177/0022167804266101.

Maidment, J., & Beddoe, L. (2012). Is social work supervision in "good heart"? A critical commentary. *Australian Social Work, 65*(2), 163–170. DOI: 10.1080/0312407X.2012.680426.

Weld, N. (2019). Facing being on shaky ground: Exploring the concept of courage through older adults' experiences of the Canterbury earthquakes. A thesis submitted in fulfilment of the requirements for the degree of Doctor of Philosophy in Social Work, the University of Auckland.

Woodard, C. R. (2010). The courage to be authentic: Empirical and existential perspectives. In C. L. S. Pury, & S. J. Lopez (Eds.), *The psychology of courage: Modern research on an ancient virtue* (pp. 109–123). Washington, DC: American Psychological Association.

8   Strengthening holistic wellbeing

Everything discussed so far in relation to applying the therapeutic function of supervision, contributes to the wellbeing of the supervisee. If existing wellbeing is present when emotional impacts occur, there will be a stronger foundation to manage these from. A holistic perspective of wellbeing identifies the key interconnected internal and external domains of wellbeing for a person, from their spiritual wellbeing through to the role of the organisations and systems they are a part of. Thinking holistically moves beyond a generalised discussion of personal 'self-care' and helps reduce the risk of a neoliberal approach where wellbeing is positioned as the responsibility of an individual. Instead, a holistic approach considers structural and contextual factors, removing the potential for individual blame and failure if a person is not well. Attending to wellbeing recognises the intertwined nature of mind and body and environment, where supporting one, supports the others.

In this chapter, a framework for holistic wellbeing is described and linked to the parasympathetic nervous system. The notion of mental fitness is explored by identifying capacities to support wellbeing that can be applied in supervision. A discussion of organisational culture that contributes to wellbeing and the importance of wellbeing for supervisors concludes the chapter.

A holistic model of wellbeing

Sir Mason Durie developed an assessment framework for Māori mental health called Te Whare Tapa Wha (the four aspects of a house). In this model, whānau (family), hinengaro (psychological – thoughts and feelings), tinana (physical) and wairua (spiritual) form the walls, roof and foundation (Durie, 1988). When all aspects of the house are

DOI: 10.4324/9781003359036-9

strong, then the house which represents a person's mental health is strong.

I applied the thinking from Te Whare Tapa Wha and developed a holistic model of wellbeing I call SPHERE. The acronym stands for Spiritual wellbeing, Physical wellbeing, a sense of Hope, Emotional wellbeing, Relational wellbeing, and a sense of Engagement (in school, social activities, work, and community). These are described in more detail in the following assessment template which can be used in supervision (Table 8.1).

Table 8.1 Sphere well-being assessment (Weld, 2014)

	Strengths	Worries	Actions
Spiritual wellbeing (sense of self-worth, identity, self-esteem, values/beliefs).			
Physical wellbeing (physical health, self-care, sleep, nutrition, exercise).			
Hope (sense of future, self-efficacy, self-belief, motivation, goals, and strengths).			
Emotional wellbeing (thoughts, feelings, mood).			
Relational wellbeing (attachment, relationships, family, friendships, supports).			
Engagement (sense of connection, belonging, activities, participation, school, work).			

A sphere is a whole and unbroken object, and in this model, all aspects of wellbeing are interconnected, with spiritual wellbeing at the heart of who we are. We can see that if one aspect of wellbeing is a bit wobbly, it can impact the other aspects. For example, if my emotional wellbeing is impacted by worry, my physical wellbeing may be impacted by not sleeping so well, then my relational wellbeing may suffer if I am tense or argumentative in my relationships which could also impact my sense of engagement at work. My sense of hope may be diminished with reduced self-efficacy, and overall, my spiritual wellbeing would suffer.

Examining our own and others' wellbeing as outlined in the template can help pinpoint areas of vulnerability and then begin to explore ways to help strengthen, restore, or rejuvenate these. I undertook the assessment with a supervisee who identified not feeling great in themselves and overall, a little low in mood. We completed the assessment together in our supervision session and they named finding it very positive in terms of reinforcing their strengths and what was working well. This in itself helped lift their mood and gave them a sense of hope moving forward. They were able to apply their other strengths to the emotional wellbeing area and make a weekly plan to intentionally do this.

When supporting a supervisee to develop actions to support their SPHERE of wellbeing, it helps to do this in a way that naturally links all six areas. An example would be arranging a weekend nature hike with a friend with a lunch in a café afterwards. In this action, physical wellbeing is addressed through movement, hope is supported by having something to look forward to, relational wellbeing is attended to by time with a friend, emotional needs are met through being able to talk and enjoy being with another person, engagement is met by being out in a social environment of a café, and overall spiritual wellbeing is supported by time in nature and being oneself. Sometimes messages around attending to wellbeing and self-care can feel complicated and overwhelming especially if someone is low on energy. The key is to make attending to self-care and wellbeing simple, interconnected, regular and as natural as possible.

Supporting the parasympathetic nervous system

A holistic approach to wellbeing brings a conscious intent to support our autonomic nervous system. The autonomic nervous system has two components – the sympathetic nervous system which activates our stress response (our fight, flight, and freeze survival response), and our parasympathetic nervous system which supports rest, repair, digestion, and calm. When our parasympathetic nervous system is engaged, we breathe slowly and deeply, and our heart rate is steady with good blood flow moving around our body and brain. Our mood is lifted and relaxed, and our digestive system functions optimally.

The way we breathe is a core contributor to whether we are engaging our sympathetic, or our parasympathetic nervous system. Awareness of our breathing throughout the day and before we go to sleep, helps us notice when we are breathing shallowly or primarily through our mouths. Clifton-Smith (2021) comments that we need to breathe "nose, low and slow" – so breathing through our noses both for inhaling and exhaling, breathing so our belly rises and extending our exhale just a little, so breathing out more. She notes that if we are inadvertently holding our breath (such as being overly focused on a computer screen) then our shoulders will be tense, and we will be sending a message to our brains to fire up our sympathetic nervous system. This can potentially increase anxiety and hence our stress response without us even being aware of it.

Generic education on breath in supervision can be very helpful, while taking care that we do not prescribe breathing practices especially if someone has an underlying respiratory or obstructed airway condition. If a supervisee is noticing they are predominantly breathing shallowly and through their mouth, they may need to seek medical advice to rule out a possible nasal or respiratory condition that might prohibit nose breathing. Developing the capacity for better breathing through a practice of pausing during the day, bringing awareness to our breath and practising 'nose, low and slow' can greatly assist with mental and physical wellbeing. Like any practice, we start gently and increase our skill levels, not force our bodies and minds into additional stress. Recognising that our breathing tells our brain whether to prepare for threat or relaxation and developing a good practice of breathing is a fundamental life skill that supports engagement of the parasympathetic nervous system. Simply extending our exhale can bring a great deal of benefit, the exhale being both an actual and a metaphoric expression of relief.

Along with the use of good breathing techniques, laughter, singing, massage (especially of the feet), humming, spending time in nature, patting an animal, being in water fasting, meditation, mindfulness, yoga, and good sleep also support the parasympathetic nervous system. When we are exploring wellbeing in supervision we can encourage all of these activities as part of a worker's weekly wellness plan.

Helping supervisee bring attention to the autonomic nervous system makes it a tangible resource and integral part of them. I was talking with a supervisee who had experienced an extremely stressful year and I asked her to imagine her nervous system and how hard it might be working. I suggested picturing her adrenal glands working on top of her kidneys and what they would look like. She said they would be shrivelled up and literally smoking! We laughed about this image (in a kind way!), and I encouraged her to identify ways to help them by supporting her parasympathetic nervous system. Being conscious of the autonomic nervous system can help increase awareness of when we may be unintentionally firing up our sympathetic nervous system, and it is helpful to explore how to apply the techniques discussed to help restore, rest, and relax and as ways to self-soothe when stressed.

Building mental fitness

The concept of 'mental fitness' helps mental health to be considered as important as physical health. To be well, we need to see both physical and mental health as equally important and make a commitment to attend to both. Just as we can decide to increase our physical fitness, we can also make a conscious decision to increase our mental fitness. With physical fitness, we might decide we need to increase our stamina or endurance, so we might do longer workouts. We might decide to increase our core strength, so we could do Pilates, or yoga. We might work on cardiovascular fitness or help build greater muscle capacity in a certain area.

Mental or psychological fitness follows the same thinking. We decide on a capacity to build or further strengthen that we know needs some attention and that will help our overall mental health fitness. Capacity building strengthens us for times ahead that may place more psychological and mental demand on us. In supervision, we can explore which areas of capacity building will help a supervisee have increased mental fitness to face challenges and stress. Along with courage and compassion, here are four capacities that we can support supervisees to build and strengthen that will contribute to greater mental health.

The capacity to relax

In a world of technology, work, and family demands, we can end up carrying significant tension in our bodies and minds. This tension may become 'normal for us' and set both our bodies and minds at a too high and unsustainable level of operating. Firstly, we need to notice this tension and identify how and where it presents itself in our bodies. A simple awareness of this might be to notice how tight we are holding our shoulders, especially if we do a lot of screen-based work. As well as having healthy sleep routines where the body and mind can recalibrate, having a daily relaxation practice helps with emotional regulation and allows the body and mind to calm and settle. This might include a structured mindfulness or meditation practice, watching fun shows, laughing with loved ones, gardening, time in nature, being in and near water, intentional muscle relaxation, reading, and gentle movement practices such as tai chi.

Building our capacity to relax so this is a daily practice helps expel and untangle tension. We can discuss these strategies in supervision and encourage supervisees to have daily relaxation practices where they get to rest and recharge. I have noticed this is especially important for supervisees who are driven and operate at a high level of 'doing' where both their minds and bodies get little chance to be relaxed and still, aside from when they are asleep.

The capacity to be in the present moment

Being present helps address anxiety, and other anticipatory emotions that are future fear-based, along with rumination or becoming lost back in past events. Writers such as Eckhart Tolle in his work on being present and in the 'now' emphasises the importance of breath, mindfulness, meditation, and nature based sensory practices that connect people to the present moment. His work reminds us that we are not our minds, and that our minds are a tool and as such they are something we can watch and observe.

Because of the discipline involved in redirecting our minds to a present focus, the practice of being present is one that most people need to build capacity in. This also helps reduce mental effort and possible distress caused by living too far out from our current reality. Along with focusing on our breath, our senses offer us an immediate way to orientate to the present by identifying what we can see, hear, taste, touch, and smell.

Being present is also about 'thought catching' where we notice our thoughts are too far out into a future that may not happen. Yes, that future might happen, and it is understandable that we want to try and be prepared for it, but it also may not, in which case our energy has been lost from enjoying life now. If using our mind to go back to a past we cannot change, and out to a future we do not fully know is causing mental distress as opposed to wellbeing, being present is the best response to this. I am very fond of the phrase "there is nothing bad happening right now" as way to ground myself and reduce future-based anxiety.

Being present also helps with building tolerance to situations of ambiguity which involve uncomfortableness of not knowing. By remaining in the present moment, we can identify what we can influence, change or plan for. Knowing what is within our circle of influence and what is not helps us refrain from trying to control the future by overly preparing in our minds. We can use our minds to pause, identify existing points of certainty, and make a small decision or take a step which will help us regain some degree of control. We can show compassion to our mind that is racing ahead to try to protect and prepare but eroding mental wellbeing in the process. Being present is about being with what is right now and the points of control we have in that.

The capacity to appreciate and be grateful

As a natural survival instinct, we are trained to notice what is not working well as this might represent danger, so building capacity of appreciation and gratitude is often a skill we all need. The theory of appreciative inquiry tells us that where we direct our thoughts is where our focus will expand so if we are focusing on what is not working well, we will more likely compound this and activate our stress arousal response. Bringing attention to what is ok and what we are grateful for is a gentler energy and one that helps us be more present.

There are a range of gratitude practices such as journaling, which involves noting down each evening five things that went well in the day that you can be grateful for. This might also include moments where we felt connected to joy which can be as simple as noticing a bird singing. A similar practice can be done to begin the day by inviting a focus on appreciation rather than worry and deficit thinking. We can encourage supervisees to notice small things that are working well during the day, or to share appreciation of something valued.

Smiling and greeting a stranger, thanking, paying forward, gifting to someone in greater need, and giving a person your full attention, all shift our energy into appreciation of what we have and what we can give. These naturally lift our mood as they also enable connection and allow us to see the good in others and in the world. To be acknowledged and to give acknowledgement, lifts our wellbeing instantly. We all need to practice redirecting our danger sensitive minds to what is good and ok in and around us and focus on seeing the beauty in the wider world of which we are a part.

The capacity to set limits

Being able to set limits in and on our work is a topic that frequently arises in supervision. Social service organisations are often under resourced, and this can cause workers to take their work home. This is evident through workers not turning their cell phones off, so being always available, responding to emails outside of work hours, and consistently working longer hours. Workers are therefore always tethered to work and this can create a low hum of pressure and anxiety that never fully abates. A supervisee may also have a high need to prove themselves and may misinterpret blurring work and home boundaries as a way of demonstrating this. The critical reflective nature of supervision means it is an ideal place to unpack this, test thinking and explore deeper motivations such as an over developed inner critic or an underlying worry about not being fully competent and having to prove oneself.

Constant giving of oneself can lead to compassion fatigue and exhaustion. Developing healthy ways to put boundaries and limits in place, such as rehearsing in supervision that skill to say no and asking for help, are ways to support the supervisee to build their capacity of setting limits. In supervision, helping a supervisee to examine what might drive a lack of setting limits and boundaries through asking curious questions helps critical reflection in a safe, non-judgemental way. They can then develop strong insight into and practices that support their mental wellbeing now and in future career roles. Simple practices such as turning work phones off unless an emergency situation requires it to be on, scheduling and taking regular leave, not going into work unwell, valuing mental health as highly as physical health (so if not feeling mentally well, it is ok to take leave just as you would if you were injured or feeling sick), having firm start and finish times each day, not taking on work beyond a person's scope of practice, and taking set breaks throughout the day, all maintain healthy boundaries and limits.

Developing these capacities, and any others a supervisee might identify to boost mental wellness and fitness, all help us build tolerance to uncertainty and difficulty. Mental and physical fitness are both deserving of our attention, and both help us endure and cope in times of strain and demand. This also makes us more nimble, flexible, responsive, and creative in our thinking rather than reactive.

Organisational culture

A supportive, and emotionally competent work culture and environment is essential to worker wellbeing. I have observed over many years of providing supervision that a significant amount of worker stress derives from the culture of the organisation they work in. To quote Sir John Kirwan, a mental health advocate in Aotearoa, New Zealand, "there's no use fixing the fish if the water is polluted". Workers particularly in large organisations are a part of complex systems with numerous parts and various impacts.

Organisations need to undertake regular and critical in-depth analysis of their culture and of the values and beliefs they hold to determine if these are still best serving those who they were set up for. An observation I would make is that organisations can move from a protective intent for clients to a protective intent for themselves resulting in increased policies, procedures and administrative demands leading to a risk adverse culture. Instead of a learning culture, there is a high compliance culture that undermines worker autonomy, creativity, and initiative.

A commitment to healthy work culture is evidenced by managers and supervisors who can engage in transformative styles of leadership, and invite and demonstrate respect, care, compassion, courage, trust, and clarity. They model and act to increase motivation, collaboration, participation, inclusiveness, openness, transparency and fairness to provide a learning culture. There is a strong commitment to developing relational capital where workers are recognised as the heart of the organisation and this is demonstrated through actively valuing workers, including inviting their participation, acknowledging, and listening to them, responding, and showing appreciation of them. A healthy workforce culture also has clear unambiguous channels of communication, including expectations of roles and responsibilities. Change is recognised and treated as a process that takes time and consideration, and care is taken to not overwhelm the workforce by a rapid and unsustainable amount of change that lacks clarity and purpose.

The Sanctuary Model developed by Dr Sandra Bloom to support a therapeutic community offers a description of an organisation committed to the wellbeing of its workforce:

> ...a strong, resilient, structured, tolerant, caring, knowledge-seeking, creative, innovative, cohesive and non-violent community where staff are thriving, people trust each other to do the right

thing, and clients are making progress in their own recovery within the context of a truly safe and connected community.

(Sanctuary Institute website)

Professor Harry Fergusson notes that unhealthy dynamics in families can also be reflected in professional systems (Ferguson, 2005). An example would be an organisation working with family violence that has internal patterns of bullying and high levels of power and control exerted on staff. Bloom suggests that it is essential that everyone in an organisation understands what toxic stress and trauma impacts look like and the behaviours that unacknowledged and unaddressed stress can cause (Bloom, 2013). This includes envisaging the future the organisation wants to have, managing the issues and losses incumbent with change and the barriers to this, developing the skills to manage interpersonal emotions around change, and addressing potential safety issues in both making and/or not making the change (Bloom, 2013, p. 286).

We also need to acknowledge that many social workers and people in social service work come to the field from their own experiences of social injustice and trauma. For those people leading a social service agency there needs to be a recognition of indirect trauma impacts, but also the likelihood that vulnerability may exist for staff from their own relational trauma histories. Managers and leaders need to be able to move deeper into therapeutic conversations and reflection with staff while retaining the boundaries of their roles. The following example below from a manager in a social service agency working with children and families who have experienced relational trauma, describes an interaction with a staff member that demonstrates this, along with their reflection about therapeutic management:

> It is always a balancing act as a manager of staff in an organization that provides therapeutic services. This is especially true when your professional background and training means you have an awareness of underlying issues that are involved when a staff member is discussing an approach or a personal reaction. Combine this with a cultivated inclination to want to dig deeper and help, alongside knowledge of vicarious trauma and a legal responsibility to keep staff emotionally safe and you can end up flexing boundaries in unforeseen ways.
>
> K was quite agitated and upset when she came to see me. She was concerned that another worker had been given an acting up role and that she and another worker had been overlooked.

From a dispassionate overview, the reaction was incongruent with reality – this was a simple 1-2 day acting up role. The 'clues' about what was going on for K were in statements about "leaving another job because of this", and about her feelings that she wanted just "to walk out and go home" there and then. She also said that this was the first time she'd talked to management about her feelings and wasn't sure whether she should have done so, or how she would be perceived as a result.

So what were my options? Perhaps refer her back to her team leader? Or briefly explain that it was not big deal and that her time would come? Or tell her she was overreacting? In the ensuing 20 minutes we covered what was behind the way she felt, which centred on being overlooked and put down in her previous role, being written off by a teacher at school, and ultimately on some child protection intervention when she was a young child. We wondered together about her reactions being a result of trauma and what help she might need, and drew a parallel with our work with adults and children as an organisation. And we found possible ways forward.

Given the inherent power differential in being a manager, it was important to honour the trust that had come my way, and acknowledge the courage that it took to talk. We haven't discussed it since, other than a brief update on who she had subsequently spoken to. But my sense is that a shift in thinking and reaction has occurred. Perhaps "therapeutic management" might be too formal a term, but helping someone who reaches out on their therapeutic journey and helping create the organisational culture and authentic relationships that allow this is, to me, and important part of being in our area of work.

(Weld, 2017, p. 96)

While a supportive and caring environment is essential, it must also hold high expectations around behaviour and professionalism. Leaders and managers should always work in ways that encourage and emphasise the resiliency of workers, knowing when and how to respond if they need greater support. Work environments need to be restorative and responsive and help workers to increase self-awareness and responsibility. If an organisation is not fully resourced to meet their contractual demands, this needs to be explored rather than a worker absorbing more and more pressure which will likely result in them possibly having to have extended time off and or even leaving. Professional supervision needs to be an established and valued part of the organisational culture, along with other restorative ways of ensuring staff feel held, heard, and cared for.

When supervising a worker who is struggling in a not so healthy work environment, it is important that as supervisors we can articulate what a healthy organisational culture can look like. By being able to do this, we can help ascertain where the organisational difficulties are and what would help. We can assist a supervisee identify their issues, reactions, and responses, and what belongs at an organisational level, as often a worker will feel that they are somehow personally failing. By using 'the problem is the problem' thinking, we will not end up colluding with supervisees in organisational blaming, but can help them differentiate what is theirs and what is a wider organisational responsibility. We can help a supervisee identify points of influence to reduce feelings of helplessness and powerlessness and to separate out the organisational factors so they do not feel responsible for wider systematic issues. It is essential though that bullying and intimidating behaviour in a workplace is never made to feel like the supervisee's responsibility, and that wider help is sought in these situations. This would include external support from a union or a professional association.

I have a clause in my supervision contract that gives me permission to speak with organisations if I am seeing difficulties presenting that pertain to organisational culture. This reads:

> If there are serious and persistent organisational concerns, the supervisee may give permission for these to be raised with the organisation by the supervisor. This recognises and addresses the collaborative partnership and responsibilities between the supervisee, organisation and supervisor.

With the ultimate focus of supervision being on supporting quality service delivery, organisational factors that seriously impact a supervisee's ability to meet this do need to be raised, with their permission. As can be seen in the above clause, this honours the partnership that is inherent in an external supervision model. When supervising a number of workers from one organisation, underlying issues and dynamics that might be impacting supervisees become evident. Finding a constructive way to raise these or to help a supervisee raise them with management, can contribute to meaningful change.

If an organisation does have longstanding problems and makes little attempt to change these, despite the issues being raised, I do support workers to see their role as potentially time limited which can help reduce their energy investment in what is happening. We can discuss what the supervisee would like to try and achieve in their remaining time, and what 'leaving well' will look like for them. I do notice worker strain reduces in this type of conversation where they can see what they could try, and to and have a plan to make the role time limited if change is not possible in a timeframe that will be effective for them. No job is worth losing your health over, and identifying and considering alternative action can assist with a supervisee's decision-making process and their wellbeing

Supervisor wellbeing

Everything that has been discussed in relational to supporting worker wellbeing applies to us as supervisors. Carroll (2014) notes that the restorative function of supervision requires supervisors to "stay strong, optimistic and resilient" and that while these can be taught to supervisees mostly they are 'caught' from supervisors (p. 74). We must have our own critically reflective supervision in place and be constantly 'taking the pulse' of our supervisory practice. Not being well in ourselves can impact this essential protected space for workers, and also send a message that may contradict what we are intending around supporting wellbeing. A distracted, tired, unwell, fatigued or stressed supervisor will run the risk of a supervisee noticing this and potentially shielding the supervisor from their own needs. Edgar Guest in the first verse of his poem 'I'd rather see a sermon' sums this up well with the line "I'd rather see a sermon than hear one any day", emphasising that actions can speak louder than words and a supervisor needs to remain mindful of this.

Supervisors need to be committed to SPHERE wellbeing practices that support mental and physical fitness. Saakvitne (2002) emphasises a "reasonable balance among work, rest and play" and "nurturing ongoing connection with others who support you in your work" (p. 447). Hearing the challenges and difficulties supervisee face, the horror they sometimes see and hear, and the distress and indirect trauma they experience requires us to monitor ourselves for signs of strain, stress, distress, emotional labour, and indirect trauma.

Supervisors are not immune to the impacts of the wider world and the joy, loss, pain, and stress that comes with living. Noticing when we may need to make arrangements to reduce work commitments to manage personal challenges is a very healthy and pro-active form of self-care. As supervisors we need to connect to places of joy, laughter, and have people in our lives who are well, healthy and doing just fine. This helps keep a balanced view and perspective of the world when we are working on a daily basis with people experiencing challenge and difficulty. Providing critically reflective supervision, especially with an intentional therapeutic component, requires focus, energy and skill. It can be tiring even when it is rewarding due to the highly focused and attentive nature of it. We need to be actively restoring and have our own wellbeing strategies in place. We need to take care around our limits and honour the supervisor relationship by keeping good boundaries. Planning an optimum number of supervision sessions in a day, keeping to time limits, having breaks in between each session so our focus is fresh and ready, and ensuring we too build in holidays and time away and partake in activities that restore and replenish us, is essential.

Summary

Supporting supervisee wellbeing and our own, requires a holistic approach that upholds the connection between our physical, emotional, mental and ultimately spiritual selves. Integrated strategies that benefit all aspects of our wellbeing reduce the possibility of self-care being singled out and added to a potentially overwhelming list of daily tasks. An integrated strategy such as supporting the parasympathetic nervous system and strengthening and building capacities to best support us in times of stress and distress makes attending to our daily wellbeing achievable. Supervisors also need to notice and question organisational culture in ways that help supervisees identify their points of influence and control. Organisations that evidence attention to building relational capital, critical reflection on their culture, and communication which is inclusive and transparent, will create environments that support worker wellbeing. Wellbeing is both a personal and an organisational responsibility, requiring both to be self-aware and willing to explore, identify, and support healthy ways of being.

References

Bloom, S. (2013). The Sanctuary Model: Changing habits and transforming the organisational operating system. In J. D. Ford, & C. A. Courtois (Eds.), *Treating complex traumatic stress disorders in children and adolescents: Scientific foundations and therapeutic models* (pp. 277–293) New York: Guilford Press.

Carroll, M. (2014). *Effective supervision for the helping professions*. London: SAGE Publications.

Clifton-Smith, T. (2021). *How to take a breath*. Auckland: Penguin NZ.

Durie, M. (1988). *Whai ora. Māori health development*. Auckland: Oxford University Press.

Ferguson, H. (2005). Working with violence, the emotions and the psycho-social dynamics of child protection: Reflections on the Victoria Climbié Case. *Social Work Education, 24*(7), 781–795. DOI: 10.1080/02615470500238702.

Saakvitne, K. W. (2002). Shared trauma: The therapist's increased vulnerability. *Psychoanalytic Dialogues, 12*, 443–449. DOI: 10.1080/10481881209348678.

Weld, N. (2014). *The Whole Sphere. Supporting wellbeing and recovery from relational trauma*. Auckland: Dunmore Publishing.

Weld, N. (2017). *E Ko te Matakahi Maire Therapeutic social work*. Stand Children Services. Wellington: Tū Māia.

Conclusion

Professional supervision provides for the integration of experiences, the building of personal and professional practice theory, the strengthening of professional identity, and the provision of a safe restorative space for those working in human service work. It attends to both professional and personal contextual factors, and its commitment to critical reflective practice invites workers to pause in their work and examine the forces and influences inherent within and around it. Professional supervision contributes to the development of both personal and professional knowledge, providing a forum for enquiry that contributes to safe practice and worker wellbeing.

As supervisors, we engage in a collaborative, relational, professional development journey with a supervisee, valuing and welcoming the opportunity to also learn about ourselves. The supervisee's safe practice and wellbeing is our priority, and one we bring a demonstrable commitment and dedication to. This is underpinned by the ultimate focus of supervision being to uphold a high-quality service delivery to some of the most vulnerable people in our societies.

The therapeutic function of supervision involves reflective, emotional, and cognitive work which reaches across a range of theories and therapy modalities, combining techniques such as a developing a coherent narrative, and the application of mindfulness, solution focused, and emotion-based questions. The therapeutic function of supervision takes place within a trusted relationship, that combines skills such as attuning, presence, and listening deeply, along with cultural humility and humbleness, requiring being comfortable in our own not knowing. The relationship itself is therapeutic, providing a mirror of how workers can engage with clients, and giving space for workers to be sustained and replenished.

Working therapeutically requires a principled and boundaried approach based on a foundation encompassing compassion and

DOI: 10.4324/9781003359036-10

courage. Vulnerability and honesty enhance insight and contribute to understanding, connection, and relationship. The locating of emotions as a vital source of information in professional supervision, allows these to be surfaced and explored, contributing to self-awareness and emotional intelligence. Applying the therapeutic function of supervision helps build the capacity to manage adversity through the continuous development of personal strength and resilience. Supervision is itself a source of resilience by helping workers best adapt and manage challenges.

Human relationships, interactions and dynamics are perhaps the most valuable place of learning for us all. While human connection can bring joy and satisfaction, disconnection can cause profound difficulty and distress. It is in relationship with others that we learn the most about ourselves, including what we have brought forward from the past and are unconsciously still working on in the present. Human service work brings us into close contact with the pain and suffering of other people and our own. In choosing this work we must be committed to critical analysis of who we are and reflective supervision that increases our consciousness. Through this we can bring the very best of ourselves to support workers manage at times the very worst of human behaviour.

Supervision is imperative in addressing the emotional impacts of social service work, providing as it does, a safe protected space where experiences are made sense of, learning found and new knowledge developed. For supervisors, the provision of professional supervision must be valued as a unique practice, not merely an extension of an existing role such as being a senior practitioner. We need to develop and grow our supervisory practice and ensure we bring the best of ourselves to it. Supervision is its own profession (Carroll, 2014), and one that deserves continued critical examination, exploration, and development.

Just as our formal mental health services will never be resourced enough for all of those who are suffering from mental distress and pain, it is not feasible that every worker experiencing emotional impacts from their work can be or should be referred to employee assistance programmes and counsellors. Professional supervision must have a therapeutic function, and supervisors should be confident to provide this.

If you have been hesitant to step into a more therapeutic function in supervision for fear of crossing a boundary into therapy, my hope is this book has shown that this will not be the case. Working from a premise of restoring and strengthening does not need the deeper dive into a person's psychological world and childhood experiences.

The therapeutic function in supervision lightly touches these, acknowledges them, connects insight from them to the work context, and returns to the professional role that is required. The supervisor always looks just past the supervisee to those they are serving, and this focus anchors the intent of professional supervision. As a supervisor we must notice any possible impacts the supervisee is experiencing and address the possible implications of these on their work first and foremost.

It is exciting to see professions such as medicine and law now accessing professional supervision and the benefits this is offering these professions. Interdisciplinary professional supervision invites learning and sharing across professions, ultimately strengthening the quality of service that is provided. This also assists with communication and collaboration in human service work through the enhancing of respect and understanding of both difference and commonality.

Work complexity and wider societal and global impacts require professional supervision to be a place of critical reflection and therapeutic restoration. The global pandemic and the ongoing economic and health impacts of this are just one feature of a world where we are increasingly required to learn to live with uncertainty. The low hum of anxiety that is present in our fragile world is best met with courage and compassion rather than with defensiveness and fear which may bring forward our survivor instinct but not necessarily our best selves. As supervisors we can step forward to meet these challenges by committing to supervisory practice that sees beyond key performance indicators and goes to the heart of human service work – humanity and service.

Professional supervision has at times, been a tacked-on requirement, an afterthought, or a cosy chat with a non-reflective description of what has been happening over the past few weeks. Professional supervision is no longer something that is nice to have now and then, or an ineffectual tick box exercise, instead it must become a core and essential part of human service work. With the articulation of the therapeutic function to attend to the emotional impacts on workers, professional supervision is further positioned as an integral source of support, learning, and knowledge.

All the very best on your supervisory journey.

Nicki Weld

Reference

Carroll, M. (2014). *Effective supervision for the helping professions*. London: Sage Publications.

Index

Note: **Bold** page numbers refer to tables and *italic* page numbers refer to figures.

Acceptance Commitment Therapy approach 101
acceptance, compassion 95–99
active experimentation 49, 52; stage of 47
Acute Stress Disorder 3, 5, 108
acute traumatic events 3
Adamson, C. 112, 114
administrative supervision *see* line management supervision
anger 62–65
anxiety 67–71
appreciation 122–123
attuning 34–36
authority 10, 21; organisational 12; power and 41, 48
autonomic nervous system 118, 119

Beddoe, L. 14, 19, 30, 47, 105
Beinart, H. 23
being present 121–122
beliefs 76–79
Benuto, L. T. 6
Berne, Eric 84
Bess, J. 77, 78
Bion, W. 56
Bloom, Sandra 124, 125
Boekankamp, D. 6
Bond, M. 13, 45, 57
boundaries 25, 27, 76, 123, 125, 129
breathing practices 119
Brown, K. 57
bullying 4, 42, 125, 127

Calhoun, L. G. 53
Callahan, J. L. 47
Carroll, M. 11, 18, 46, 57, 66, 67, 128
Carter, M.-A. 89
Casement, P. 16
chronic stress *see* long-term stress
chronic trauma 4, 5
Clifton-Smith, T. 119
clinical supervision 9–12
Clohessy, S. 23
Cognitive Affective Supervisory Approach 58
coherent narrative: connect to strengths and existing resiliency 50–52; development of 53; inaccurate thoughts, exploring of 49–50; moving forward 52–54; reflective learning processes 46–49
compassion 89, 103; anchor to core motivation 94–95; defined as 89–91; develop acceptance, understanding and connection 95–99; emotional regulation 92–94; *vs.* empathy 93; self-awareness 91–92; self-compassion and self-forgiveness 99–102
compassion fatigue 6, 80, 123; exposure of 5
compassion satisfaction 6
Complex Post-Traumatic Stress Disorder (CPTSD) 4
connection, compassion 95–99
conscious decision 107–109

Cornell, A.W. 59
counter-transference 80–83
courage 105; application to
  supervision 108–109; defined
  as 106–107; process model of
  108, *108*; questions to connect
  109–110; stage of 107–108
CPTSD *see* Complex Post-Traumatic
  Stress Disorder (CPTSD)
Cree, V. 2, 56–57
critical reflection 15, 19, 24, 31, 46,
  54, 102, 123, 129, 133
critical thinking 16, 107
cultural humility 39–42
Cummings, C. 6

Davys, A. 14, 19, 47
depression 1, 74, 81, 97
Dewane, C. 77–80
Dillon, R. S. 100
disappointment 60–62
distress 3, 4, 7, 25, 45, 59, 60, 108;
  for supervisees 76
distress tolerance 92–93
Dolezal, L. 65, 66
Doty, J. R. 97
the drama triangle 84–86
Durie, Sir Mason 116

Edwards, J. 77, 78
emotional based questions 37–38
emotional containment: supervision
  as space for 56–59; work of 58
emotional distress 25
emotional experiences 6, 12, 60, 82,
  90, 93
emotional exploration 58
emotional expression 58, 74, 94
emotional intelligence 132
emotional labour 1, 2, 5–7, 58, 97
emotionally sensitive supervision 59
emotional management 21–22
emotional pressure, of working 2
emotional regulation 24, 92–94,
  107, 120
emotional responses 39, 49, 57, 59
emotional wellbeing 117, **117**, 118
emotions 56, 132; anger 62–65;
  anxiety 67–71; disappointment
  60–62; grief 71–74; overwhelm

59–60; shame 65–67;
  suppressed 59
empathy 90, 103; compassion *vs.* 93
empathy fatigue 6
The Empowerment Dynamic 84–85
Enright, R. 99
exercise 63, 70, 87
exhaustion 60, 113, 123
experiential learning 33
externalising 86, 87, 95
external professional supervision 17
external reflection 46

Fairfield, Mark 94
fear 91, 105, 108
Ferguson, H. 16, 125
Field, R. 57
Flowers, B. S. 32
focus groups 81
formative function, professional
  supervision 19
Francis, A. P. 89
Frazier, P. 68
frustration 61, 63; mixture of anger
  and 64

generic education, on breath 119
Gibson, M. 65, 66
GRAPE process 47
gratitude 122–123
Gray, I. 57
Great Wars 3
grief 71–74
grit 105, 110–112
group supervision 9
guilt 101–102

Hadfield, M. 2, 56–57
Halifax, Joan 106
Hallett, S. 2, 56–57
Harkness, D. 18
harm 4, 5, 17, 26, 94, 95, 101
Hawkins, P. 7, 11, 13, 20, 24, 46,
  57, 78
healing 22, 95
healthy workforce culture 124
Hisaka, R. 6
historical/multigenerational trauma,
  impact of 4
Hochschild, A. R. 1, 56

Holland, S. 13, 45, 57
honesty 132; and transparency 32
Hook, J. N. 40
human relationships 76, 132
human service work 131, 133;
    compassion 94; courage 105, 106;
    emotional impacts of 7
human service worker 1, 4

inaccurate thoughts, exploring of
    49–50
indirect trauma 5–7, 56, 125
individual supervision 9, 10
Ingham, Harrington 39
Ingham, R. 11, 58, 59
interdisciplinary professional
    supervision 133
interdisciplinary supervision 13–15
internal supervision 9
interprofessional supervision,
    principles of 14
irritation 62–64, 98
Itzhaky, H. 20, 21
Itzhaky, T. 20, 21

Jaworski, J. 32
Johari window 39, 77

Kadusshin, A. 18
Kaitiakitanga approach 11–12, 16
Kellogg, M. 5
kindness 78; and care 103; self-
    directed 101; and sensitivity 66;
    and understanding 99
Kirwan, Sir John 124
Knapman, J. 20
Kolb, D. 33
Kolb experiential learning cycle
    (1984) 46–49, 52
Krupka, Z. 24

Levenson, J. 30
line management supervision 9, 10
listening 36–37
long-term stress 2
Luft, Jospeh 39

Maidment, J. 105
Māori concept, of 'Wātea' 33
Maté, Gabor 60–61

McMahon, A. 20, 24
meaning 61, 73
mental fitness 120; capacity to
    appreciate and be grateful
    122–123; capacity to be in present
    moment 121–122; capacity to
    relax 120–121; capacity to set
    limits 123
mental toughness 111
Miller, B. 2, 6, 95
mindfulness 82, 119, 121, 131
"model of mind" 95
Morrison, F. 2, 56–57
Morrison, T. 18, 20
motivations 107; anchor to core
    94–95
Munro, E. 100

natural disasters 3, 112
negative experiences 53, 54, 78
negative social media 68
negative thoughts 111
Neimeyer, R. 72
Ng, A. K. T. 41
Nickson, A. M. 89
non-judgemental attitude 95
normative function, professional
    supervision 19
nurses, criteria checklist for 13

O'Donoghue, K. 12, 25, 31, 41
'one word answer' 38
openness 32, 40
ordering principles 77–78
organisational blaming 127
organisational culture 124–128
'othering' 91
overwhelm 59–60

Page, S. 20, 21
parallel process 80–83
parasympathetic nervous system
    118–120
Pasifika cultures 41
Paulin, V. 11
Payne, C. 18
peer supervision 9
people-management processes 10
persistent rumination 66
personality 76–79

personal self 76, 77
physical fitness 120, 123, 128
physical/psychological safety 3, 4,
    62, 107
physical wellbeing 117, **117**, 118
Post Traumatic Growth (PTG)
    53, 54
Post-Traumatic Stress Disorder
    (PTSD) 3–4
power 41; and authority 41, 48;
    incorrect attribution of 50
presence 32–34
'problem is the problem not the
    person' 86–87
Proctor, B. 18, 19
professional accommodation
    syndrome 2
professional dangerousness 1, 17, 69
professional identity 13, 14, 19
professional self 76, 77
professional supervision 1, 7, 9,
    11–13, 30, 77, 126–127, 131–133;
    formative function 19; functions
    of 18–20; normative function 19;
    restorative function 19, 20; roles
    in 15–18
psychological first aid 45
psychological fitness *see* mental
    fitness
PTG *see* Post Traumatic Growth
    (PTG)
PTSD *see* Post-Traumatic Stress
    Disorder (PTSD)
pursuer/withdrawer dynamics 85

Reflective Learning Model 47
reflective learning processes 17,
    46–49
reflective practice 46, 131
reflective space 16, 25
reflective supervision 107, 129
relational dynamics 76, 87–88;
    counter-transference and parallel
    process 80–83; personality, beliefs,
    and values 76–79; 'problem is the
    problem not the person' 86–87;
    transactional analysis 83–86; use
    of self-disclosure 79–80
relational skills 42–43; attuning
    34–36; cultural humility 39–42;

enabling vulnerability 37–39;
    listening 36–37; presence 32–34
relational space 41, 43; for cultural
    difference 40
relational trauma 65, 84, 125
relational wellbeing 117, **117**, 118
relaxation practice 120–121
resilience/resiliency 50–52, 105,
    112–114
restorative function, professional
    supervision 19, 20
Richards, M. 18
Rodgers, A. 33
Rossomando, T. 97
Rotter, J. B. 78
Ruch, G. 2, 16, 56–58

Saakvitne, K. W. 128
safe practice 20, 59, 131
safety: acceptance and 35;
    organisational 9; physical/
    psychological 3, 4, 62, 107; in
    supervision 58; wellbeing and 17,
    32, 69, 71, 103
The Sanctuary Model 124
Schamess, G. 23, 34, 76, 80, 81
Scharmer, O. C. 32
Schon, D. 46
secondary trauma *see* indirect
    trauma
secondary traumatic stress (STS) 5,
    6, 106, 108
self-actualised people 109–110
self-awareness 71, 74, 87, 90, 91–92,
    103, 126, 132
self-blame 49, 50, 101
self-care 41, 116, 118, 128
self-compassion 89, 99–103
self-disclosure, use of 79–80
self-forgiveness 99–102
self-knowledge 80, 87, 110
self-reproach 100
self, utilisation of 80
Senge, P. 32
sense of engagement 117, **117**, 118
sense of hope 117, **117**, 118
Seppala, E. 97
Seven Eyed model of supervision 11
sexual abuse accommodation
    syndrome 65

shadow motives 78
shame 65–67
"shame anxiety" 65
shame sensitivity 66
shell shock 3–4
Shohet, R. 7, 13, 18, 46, 57, 78
short-term stress 2
Singer, J. 6
social connectedness 97
social service organisations 123
social service work 56, 57, 125;
  emotional impacts of 132;
  relational nature of 77
social service workers 6
societal stressors 51
SPHERE wellbeing 117, **117**,
  118, 128
spiritual wellbeing 116, 117, **117**
Sprang, G. 2, 6, 95
stage of active experimentation 47
strength-based practice principle 86
stress 2, 7; emotional impacts of
  12; long-term 2; short-term 2; for
  supervisees 76
stress response 62, 68, 70, 118, 119
STS *see* secondary traumatic
  stress (STS)
Sudbery, J. 80
suffering 60, 89; exposure of 5
Summit, Roland 65
supervisees: autonomy of 16; choice
  of supervisor 31; emotional
  containment for 25; entered
  vulnerability 39; external
  reflection 46; personal dynamics
  of 24; positive qualities of
  67; stress and distress for 76;
  wellbeing of 17
supervision 3, 132; coherent
  narrative in 53; ethical
  considerations 26–27; to explore
  anxiety 70; goals of 21; grit 111;
  professional 7; reflective learning
  processes 46; resilience 112;
  safe relational space for cultural
  difference 40; safety in 58; single
  page recording sheet in 51; as
  space for emotional containment
  56–59; supportive function of 18;
  therapeutic and therapy boundary
20–25; therapeutic function of
  7–9, 131–133; types of 9–13
Supervision Session Pyramid 47–48
supervisors 9, 89, 131; with cultural
  humility 40; role of 12
supervisor wellbeing 128–129
supervisory relationship 42–43;
  developing of 30–32
supervisory space 18, 22
suppressed emotions 59
surface acting 2, 63, 89

Tedeschi, R. G. 53
Te Whare Tapa Wha 116–117
'therapeutikos' 22
Tolle, Eckhart 70, 121
transactional analysis 83–86
transference 80–83
transferential dynamics, self-
  identification of 83
transparency 27, 32; honesty and 32;
  openness and 40
trauma 7; exposure of 5; personal
  histories of 6; relational 65, 84,
  125; social injustice and 125
Trauma Focused Cognitive
  Behaviour Therapy 45
trauma narrative 45, 96
trust 36, 37, 97
Tsui, M.-s. 41
Turney, D. 16, 58

unconscious decision 107
'unconscious ordering principles' 77
understanding, compassion 95–99
'U' theory 32–33, 53

values 76–79
vicarious trauma 5, 6, 125
Vîşcu, L. 47
vulnerability 118, 132; enabling
  37–39

Watkins, C. E. 47
Webber-Dreadon, E. 11
Weld, Nicki 58, 69, 71, 72, 73, 76,
  107, 110, **117**, 126, 133
wellbeing 70–71, 116, 129; holistic
  model of 116–118, **117**; mental
  fitness 120–123; organisational

culture 124–128; parasympathetic nervous system 118–120; and safety 17, 32, 69, 71, 103; supervisor wellbeing 128–129

Winter, K. 2, 56–57

The Wisdom of Trauma (Maté) 60–61

Woodard, C. R. 109

work/working: complexity 133; emotional impacts of 12; emotional pressure of 2; in human service work 131; with shame 66

Wosket, V. 20, 21

For Product Safety Concerns and Information please contact our EU
representative GPSR@taylorandfrancis.com
Taylor & Francis Verlag GmbH, Kaufingerstraße 24, 80331 München, Germany

www.ingramcontent.com/pod-product-compliance
Lightning Source LLC
Chambersburg PA
CBHW071418290326
41932CB00046B/2398

9 7 8 1 0 3 2 4 1 6 3 6 6